Anna Barwi

Still Here, Still You:
Understanding Life After Spinal Cord Injury

A Straight-Talking Guide for Families, Carers and the Newly Injured

find me on instagram

@THOSEWHODARETOCARE

Copyright © 2025 by Anna Barwinek
All rights reserved.
No portion of this book may be reproduced in any form without written permission from the publisher or author, except as permitted by U.S. copyright law.

To one soul, now gone, whose strength, humour and heart left a mark I will carry forever. This book is, in part, for you - for your courage, your fight, inspiration and the quiet legacy you leave behind.

And to Sam
Thank you for being the calm and steady presence through laughter and tears, long days and late nights, and the kind of person who never stopped showing up. Your strength, integrity and kindness shaped me as a carer and helped me find my feet when it felt impossible to move forward.

You can give without loving, but you can never love without giving.

Victor Hugo

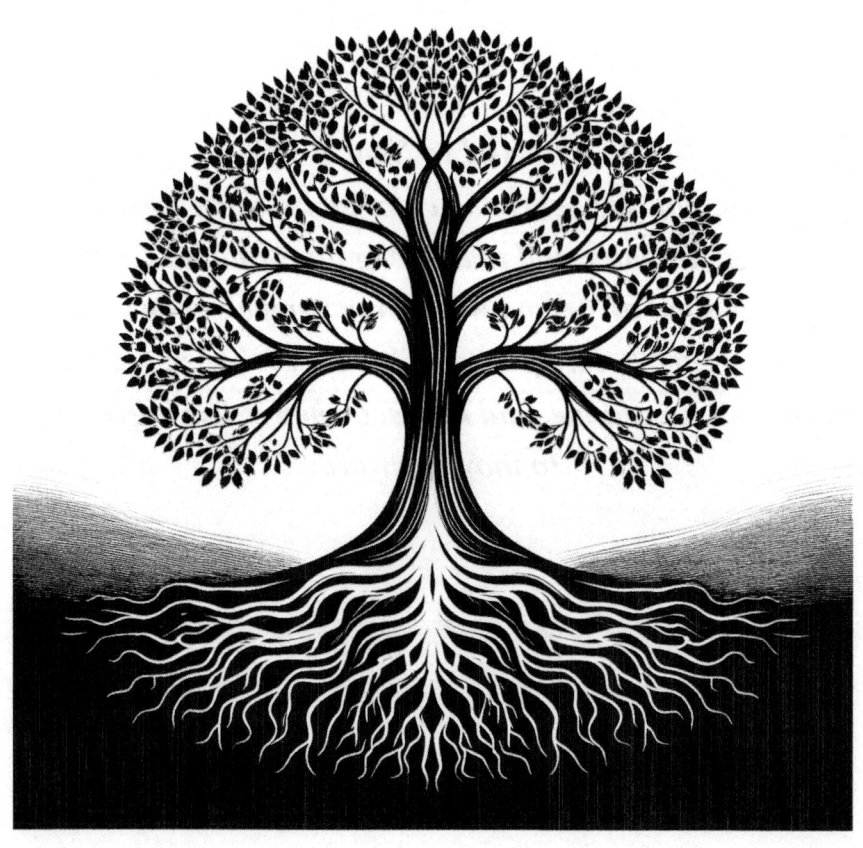

Table of Content

A Letter to You: Before You Begin
Page 7

Introduction
Page 9

Chapter 1: Understanding Spinal Injury
Page 11

Chapter 2: The First Days and Weeks
Page 18

Chapter 3: The New Normal
Page 27

Chapter 4: Understanding Care Needs
Page 32

Chapter 5: Choosing and Organising Care
Page 46

Chapter 6: Coming Home - Adapting Your Home and Building Independence
Page 57

Chapter 7: Daily Routines and Rebuilding Confidence at Home
Page 65

Chapter 8: Risks and How to Manage Them
Page 71

Chapter 9: Learning, Purpose, and Returning to Work
Page 98

Chapter 10: Emotional Wellbeing, Relationships, and Intimacy After Spinal Injury
Page 104

Chapter 11: Parenting and Family Life After Spinal Injury
Page 114

Chapter 12: Finding Support, Building Community, and Staying Connected
Page 120

Chapter 13: Travel and Freedom
Page 127

Travel Preparation Checklist
Page 134

Chapter 14: Life After Injury - Purpose, Resilience and Living Fully
Page 136

Chapter 15: Planning for the Future
Page 143

Closing Words: A Letter of Gratitude and Hope
Page 150

Resources and Further Support
Page 152

A Letter to You: Before You Begin

Dear Reader

Before you turn the page, I want to thank you for picking up this book. Whether you are reading it as a partner, a parent, a sibling, a friend or as someone living with a spinal cord injury yourself, I am glad you are here.

This book was written from a place of deep respect. Respect for the people I have supported, for the families who have stood beside them, and for every quiet act of courage I have witnessed in hospital wards, living rooms, care plans and uncertain moments. I have seen what spinal injury does. The fear, the grief, the strength it takes to wake up in a body that no longer feels like your own. I have seen what it takes and I have also seen what it gives. The humour, the friendships, the perspective, the depth.

Nothing in this book is here to sugar coat the truth. This is not a story about everything working out perfectly. But it is a reminder that even when life changes in ways you never expected - it can still hold love, laughter, meaning and moments that matter.

You do not need to have all the answers. None of us do. You may read every word or dip into the chapters that speak most to your situation. However you choose to read it, I hope you find something here that offers clarity, comfort, or courage.

This book was never just about facts. It is built on years of lived experience - on early mornings, long nights, routines, setbacks, and everyday victories. On cups of tea and conversations that stayed with me. It is as personal as it is practical. And I hope it will remind you that even in the hardest chapters, you still get to write your story.

If you ever wish to reach out - to ask a question, share your story, or speak to someone who understands - you are welcome to email me at:
talktoanna@pm.me

I cannot promise instant answers, but I promise to read what you write with care.

You are not alone.
You are not broken.
And you are not without hope.

With warmth, respect and belief in you
Anna

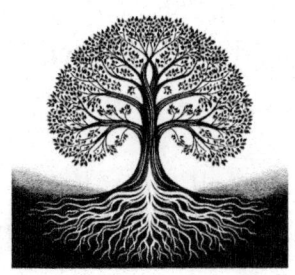

Introduction

This Is Not the End

If you are reading this book, your life has likely just changed - suddenly and dramatically. Someone you love has sustained a spinal cord injury, and now everything feels uncertain. The hospital is full of unfamiliar terms. The future looks nothing like the one you pictured. You are likely overwhelmed, frightened and wondering what comes next.

This book is for you.

My name is Anna, and for the past nineteen years, I have worked in a field that is full of misconceptions, often overlooked, yet life-changing - spinal injury care. I never set out to work in this profession. When I moved to the UK, no one would hire me without experience, despite my background. So I applied for a live-in care position - thinking it would be six months at most, just something to get started. Eight days later, I completed my training, terrified I had overestimated myself. But less than three months into the job, I fell in love with it. Nineteen years later, I still am.

This work is demanding - not just physically, but emotionally. You become someone's hands, legs, advocate, counsellor, and confidante. You hold their dignity, safety and wellbeing in your hands. You witness heartbreak and unimaginable resilience.

You learn to listen more than you speak, to act without ego, and to keep showing up - even on the hardest days.

I have spent the last nineteen years caring for, supporting and walking alongside people with spinal injuries. I have helped them navigate everything from emergency hospital stays to day-to-day routines at home. I have seen the darkest moments - and I have seen people laugh again, love again, find purpose, travel the world and adapt in extraordinary ways.

So no, this is not just a job. It is a calling. I have been told I am "just a carer," but I stand tall in my profession. I am highly skilled and deeply committed. I have studied, trained, and poured my heart into supporting people through some of the most difficult moments of their lives. And in return, I have been gifted with perspective, connection, and countless moments of joy.

That is why I wrote this book.

This book is not just a list of medical facts or a folder full of checklists. It is a companion. A guide for those first terrifying days and the long road that follows. It is here to make things clearer when nothing feels clear. You will find practical information about spinal injury care - what is needed, what to watch out for, what support is out there. But you will also find something else: the human side. The quiet realities, the fears families do not always say out loud, the things I have learned from the brave and resilient people I have had the privilege to care for.

This is not just a guide to spinal injury - it is a companion for families and loved ones who are suddenly facing the unknown.

You will find honest, practical advice about what to expect, how to plan care, how to avoid risks, and how to build a new kind of life. But you will also find hope, compassion and a reminder that you are not alone.

Spinal injury changes everything. But life does not end here. There is still so much love, laughter and purpose ahead. You may not see that yet and that is okay. I have seen it, many times over. And I will help you see it too. I hope what is inside these pages helps you find your footing in this new world, one step at a time, in your own way and in your own time.

You do not need to have all the answers right now. My hope is that this book helps you feel more prepared, more supported and a little less alone as you learn to live well in this new reality. This book is for family members, partners, friends, and yes, even for those who sustained spinal cord injury. It is for anyone facing the reality of spinal injury and wondering how to live in this unfamiliar version of life. Because that is what it is - not the end, but the beginning of something different. Life will not go back to how it was before. But it will go on.

And there is so much life left to live

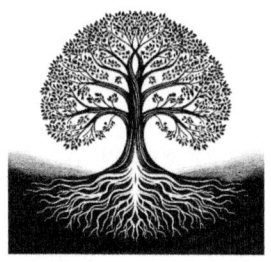

Chapter 1: Understanding Spinal Injury

What It Means and What Comes Next

When someone you love sustains a spinal cord injury, the words alone can feel like a wave crashing over you. It is a medical term that carries a lifetime of implications. But like everything else in life, understanding it begins with small, manageable pieces.
This chapter is your starting point.

What Is a Spinal Cord Injury (SCI)?

The spinal cord is a thick band of nerves running from the brain down the back. It is responsible for sending messages between the brain and the rest of the body. A spinal cord injury (SCI) happens when that cord is damaged - through trauma, illness, or disease - disrupting the flow of signals.

The result? Loss of movement, sensation, or both, below the point of injury. The extent depends on the level of injury and whether it is complete or incomplete.

Levels of Injury

The spine is made up of sections:
- Cervical (neck) C1- C7
- Thoracic (upper back) T1 – T12
- Lumbar (lower back) L1 – L5
- Sacral (base of the spine) S1- S4

The higher the injury, the more of the body is affected. For example:

A **cervical injury** may affect both arms and legs (called tetraplegia or quadriplegia):

C1-C3 nerves: Control head and neck movement, enabling basic functions like turning, tilting and nodding the head. They are also essential for stabilising the head's position.
C4 nerves: Assist with breathing by controlling the diaphragm and contribute to shoulder movement, enabling shrugging and basic arm positioning.
C5 nerves: Influence muscles in the shoulders and upper arms, allowing for shoulder rotation, lifting the arms and initiating elbow flexion.
C6 nerves: Critical for wrist extension, allowing for controlled hand positioning and some forearm movement.
C7 nerves: Enable elbow extension and some finger movements, playing a role in grasping, releasing and fine motor skills.

A **thoracic** or **lumbar** injury may affect only the legs (paraplegia), leaving arm and hand function intact.

T1 nerves: Provides motor and sensory function to the hands and fingers. It contributes to fine motor skills, dexterity, and coordination, essential for tasks like gripping, writing, and manipulating small objects.

T2-T5 nerves: Affect the muscles of the upper chest. They help stabilise the rib cage, support breathing, and help in movements like lifting or pushing. Proper function in this region is vital for maintaining respiratory health and upper body strength.

T6-T8 nerves: Influence the chest and upper abdominal muscles. They play a role in deeper breathing by engaging the diaphragm and upper abdominal muscles, contributing to core stability and balance. This section also helps with posture and protects the spine during movement.

T9-T12 nerves: Control the lower abdominal muscles, which are key to maintaining posture, protecting internal organs, and aiding in movements such as bending, twisting, and coughing. Proper abdominal muscle function is essential for core strength, which supports activities like standing, sitting, and physical exertion.

L1 and L2 nerves: Control hip bending and flexing, critical for walking and sitting.

L3 nerves: Enables knee straightening, important for standing and maintaining stability.

L4 nerves: Allows the foot to bend upward (dorsiflexion), aiding in balance and movement.

L5 nerves: Supports toe extension, necessary for precise movements like walking on uneven surfaces.

Complete vs Incomplete Injury

- A complete injury means there is no sensory or motor function below the injury site.
- An incomplete injury means some signals still get through - there may be partial sensation, movement, or both.

The exact outcome is unique to each person. And sometimes it takes weeks or even months to know what recovery, if any, is possible. Do not try to compare - two people with the same level of injury will face completely different outcome, there will be different abilities and motor skills preserved, recovered, retrained. We are all different, so please do not try to compare your loved one's injury to other people's.

The First Few Days: A Whirlwind of Information

The immediate aftermath of a spinal injury is chaotic. Families are often given a lot of clinical information - scans, medical terms, risk assessments - but very little emotional or practical guidance. You may feel overwhelmed by specialists, machines and fear.

This period is often spent in ICU or a trauma ward, stabilising the person and preventing further injury. There may be surgery to relieve pressure or realign the spine. You will hear terms like "spinal shock," "neurogenic bladder" and "autonomic dysreflexia" - unfamiliar words that will soon become part of daily life.

It is okay if it does not all make sense yet. You are not expected to become an expert overnight.

Grieving What is Lost

Let us name something important: spinal injury is not just a physical trauma - it is an emotional one. There is a grief process. And not just for the injured person, but for the people who love them.

You might grieve the life you had imagined, the things you thought would be easy, the roles that may now shift in your relationship. These are valid, heavy emotions. There is no timeline for them. What matters is that you acknowledge them - and that you find support for yourself, not just for your loved one.

That support might come from family and close friends. But it often needs to go further than that.

Reach out. Speak to a counsellor or therapist who understands trauma, loss, or caring roles. Find a support group or online community. Peer support - connecting with others who have walked this path - can be especially powerful. They will not just understand what you are going through; they will know what helped them, what did not, and how to hold space for what you are feeling.

You will need that space. Because however strong you are, you cannot pour from an empty cup. You will need somewhere to talk, to cry, to vent. You will need people who will not flinch at your honesty. If you try to carry it all in silence, burnout will creep in, quietly, but quickly.

Support is not a luxury. It is a lifeline. You deserve it just as much as the person you are standing beside. And remember, one day you will be on the other side of this - stronger, steadier and this will not feel so raw. When that time comes, you will be able to support someone else, helping them find their way through the same life changing challenges you have lived.

The Truth About Prognosis

One of the hardest things to accept early on is this: doctors often will not give a clear prognosis. That is not because they are hiding something, but because recovery from spinal injury is unpredictable. The nervous system is complex, and every injury, and every person is different. What you may hear is this: "Let's wait and see."

In some ways, this is both terrifying and hopeful. There are people who regain more than expected. And there are those who do not recover in the way they or their families hoped. But even in those cases, people learn to live meaningful, joyful, independent lives - with the right support and mindset.

What You Can Do Right Now

- Ask questions - even the "silly" ones. Clarity is power.
- Take breaks when you need them. This is a marathon, not a sprint.
- Find someone to talk to - a nurse, a counsellor, a trusted friend.
- Write things down - appointments, terms, questions. Your mind is doing a lot.

And remember you are not alone. Millions of families around the world have walked this path. This is not the future you planned, but it can still be a good future.

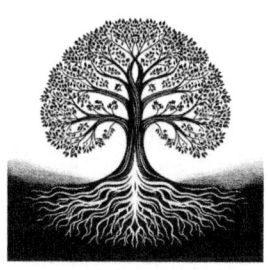

Chapter 2: The First Days and Weeks

What to Expect in Hospital and Early Recovery

The early days after a spinal injury are some of the most intense and emotionally charged moments a family can experience. Everything feels urgent. There are doctors coming and going, machines beeping, and decisions being made that you barely have time to process. Sleep is a blur, fear is constant, and you may feel like you are living minute to minute.

This chapter is here to help you slow down and understand what is happening, both in the hospital room and within yourself.

The Hospital Phase: Stabilisation and Survival

The first priority after a spinal injury is preserving life and stabilisation. Depending on the injury, your loved one may be in the ICU (intensive care unit) or high dependency unit for close monitoring.

The main goals during this phase are:
- Preventing further damage to the spinal cord
- Managing other injuries (head trauma, internal bleeding, broken bones)
- Reducing swelling around the spine
- Maintaining stable blood pressure, breathing, and organ function

You may hear terms like:
- Spinal shock – a temporary loss of function and reflexes below the injury, making it hard to assess long-term damage early on.
- Ventilated patient – high spinal injuries (especially in the cervical region) may affect the ability to breathe independently.
- Log-rolling – a careful technique used for moving the patient without twisting the spine.
- Neuro obs – neurological observations taken regularly to monitor brain and spinal cord function.

It can feel like everything is out of your hands. And in many ways, it is. But knowing what is happening, and why, can help you feel more in control.

Meeting the Medical Team

You will likely be introduced to a lot of professionals. It is okay if you cannot remember all their names at first. Each of them plays a role in your loved one's care:

- Consultants – lead doctors overseeing treatment.
- Neurosurgeons/Orthopaedic surgeons – may be involved if surgery is needed.
- Nurses – provide 24/7 care and are often your most immediate source of updates and support.
- Physiotherapists (PTs) – begin gentle movement and respiratory care, even in ICU.
- Occupational Therapists (OTs) – assess function and start thinking about future independence.

- Speech and Language Therapists (SLTs) – may help with communication or swallowing if needed.
- Psychologists or counsellors – sometimes offered for emotional support.

You are allowed to ask questions. You are entitled to understand the plan. And if something does not make sense, ask again.

Emotions: The Rollercoaster

Families often go through a huge emotional crash in these first days. You might be in fight - or - flight mode, handling practical tasks and relaying news to others. And then, suddenly, you will break down in a hospital corridor or find yourself crying in the car. This is normal.

You might also feel:

- Guilt ("Why didn't I do something?")
- Anger ("Why did this happen to us?")
- Helplessness
- Hope and despair, sometimes within the same hour

There is no right way to feel. But you do need space to feel it. Even if that means stepping away from the bedside. Your loved one needs you strong and steady - but that does not mean emotionally numb. You need to look after yourself and no, you do not have to be brave and strong 100% of the time. If the hospital has family liaison teams, social workers, or therapists, ask for a conversation. Early emotional support makes a huge difference.

Rehabilitation: Planning the Next Step

Once your loved one is medically stable, talk will begin about rehabilitation. Depending on your location and healthcare system, this may involve transfer to a spinal injury unit or neuro-rehab centre.

Rehab is where the real work begins:
- Physio for muscle strength, posture, and breathing
- Occupational therapy to relearn everyday tasks
- Assessments for mobility aids and assistive equipment
- Emotional support and psychological adjustment

Rehab can last weeks or months - and it is often a slow, frustrating process. But it is also where many families begin to rebuild hope. You will meet others on the same path, and you will start to learn what life with spinal injury can look like.

What You Can Do Right Now

- Start a notebook: Record updates, questions, medical terms and milestones. This becomes an invaluable reference.
- Be present, but pace yourself: Staying strong for someone does not mean burning yourself out.
- Learn the basics: Start asking about your loved one's injury level, whether it is complete/incomplete, and what that might mean.
- Ask about rehab early: If a spinal unit is an option, inquire about waiting lists and referrals.
- Prepare for change: Your routines, home life, and relationships may shift - but you are not powerless in the face of it.

A Note on Hope

Families often ask: "Will they ever walk again?"
And the truth is: sometimes yes, often no. But walking is not the only measure of a life worth living. I have supported people who have travelled, built families, run businesses, and found joy again - without ever walking again.

So, if you are searching for hope, start here: this is not the end. It is the beginning of a different life. And it can still be a good one

Rehabilitation: A New Beginning

Rehabilitation is not just about movement. It is where rebuilding begins - physically, emotionally, and practically. Once your loved one is medically stable, the next step is often a stay in a specialist spinal rehabilitation unit, which might be part of a larger hospital or an entirely separate facility. These centres are designed to help patients learn to live well with a spinal cord injury, no matter their level of ability.

In rehab, everything shifts from survival to living.

You may be surprised at how much is covered in these units:
- Physiotherapy helps with strengthening muscles, improving posture, and learning how to move safely again.
- Occupational therapy helps with relearning daily tasks like dressing, using the toilet, and preparing food.
- Bowel and bladder management is taught with dignity, patience, and practical tools.

- Psychological support is often available, because adjusting mentally is as important as the physical side.
- Patients will also start learning to use equipment - manual or powered wheelchairs, hoists, standing frames - and building the confidence to use them independently when possible or to instruct his future care team on what works and how they want to parts of their routine completed.
- And finally, they learn and memorise their whole care routine, so when discharged there will be no hesitation in guiding their carers through the daily routine.

I want to add that families usually learn right alongside the person with the injury. In fact, I have not met a single client whose loved ones did not know their care routine inside out. Over the years, I have witnessed more than a few moments where that knowledge made all the difference - stepping in when the person could not speak for themselves, keeping things safe, calm and familiar.

It is vital that the person with the injury understands their own care routine - not just to build confidence, but so they can clearly guide carers once they are home. But there are times, especially during illness or fatigue, when someone else has to step in and carry that knowledge for them.

I remember being in hospital with one of my clients. In the bed next to him was another young man who was very unwell, unable to speak up or manage his care. He did not have a carer with him. He had his mum. And she knew every detail of his routine. I watched as she calmly, gently, but firmly advocated for him. She guided the nurses on how to reposition him, how to manage his bowel care safely, how to avoid triggers for autonomic dysreflexia. No one had formally trained her, she had learned it all out of love and necessity. Her presence kept him safe, comfortable, and cared for when he could not direct things himself.

That moment has never left me. It was a reminder that care often extends beyond professionals and that the knowledge and strength families carry is just as essential.

The length of stay in rehab can vary depending on the injury, the patient's goals and availability of services. It is rarely short. But that is because it is vital.

One of my clients, a man with a high level spinal injury, spent his rehab at the Salisbury Spinal Centre - a place known not just for its medical expertise but for its spirit. He told me about a long corridor there, set on an uphill bend. It became something of an unspoken rite of passage among the patients. The quiet goal was this: to make it, unassisted, to the top of that corridor in your wheelchair. For him, who had a powered chair, it was a bit of a cheat - once he had mastered his joystick control, he proudly zipped up the hill and teased the nurses that he was "ready to go home." But for many, that corridor symbolised much more than mobility. It was a personal mountain. Reaching the top meant strength, independence and a glimpse of the life that still lay ahead.

Discharge Is not the End of Support

One of the biggest fears families have is: "What happens when we go home? Are we on our own?"
The answer is - no. Discharge from rehab is not the end of care. In fact, most spinal injury centres consider their patients to be lifelong members of their service. That means your loved one is

not just being "sent off", they are stepping into the next phase, backed by a network of professionals who remain just a phone call away.

Most spinal units have:
- An outreach team - specially trained spinal nurses who can advise over the phone or visit patients at home if any issues arise.
- A specialist tissue viability team - experts in preventing and treating pressure sores, a serious risk for many SCI patients.
- Continued access to physiotherapists, urology clinics and wheelchair services.
- Some also offer peer support programmes, where former patients offer guidance and emotional support to those newly injured.

If something changes - an infection, equipment issue, emotional crisis - there are people who know exactly what to do. You are never left to figure it out on your own.

There are also incredible charities dedicated to supporting those affected by spinal injury and they can make a world of difference.

The Spinal Injuries Association (SIA) is a lifeline for many, offering expert advice, legal and welfare support, advocacy and a listening ear from people who truly understand. Whether you need help navigating care, accessing funding, or simply want to speak with someone who has been through it all - they are there.

The Back Up Trust is another powerful source of encouragement and connection. They help people with spinal injuries rebuild confidence, discover new interests, and reconnect with the world. From wheelchair skills training to life coaching and adventurous group challenges (including skiing, abseiling, or even climbing Mount Snowdon) their work shows that life after injury can still be full of excitement, exploration, and community.

Do not be afraid to reach out. These organisations exist because you matter and because no one should have to face this journey alone.

Spinal injury changes everything. But life does not end here. There is still so much love, laughter, and purpose ahead. You may not see that yet - and that is okay. You do not need to have all the answers right now. My hope is that this book helps you feel more prepared, more supported, and a little less alone as you begin to understand this new way of living.

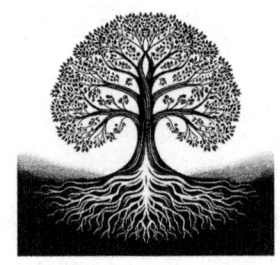

Chapter 3: The New Normal

Adjusting to Life After Spinal Injury

There is a moment, usually sometime after hospital discharge or midway through rehab, when the pace slows and reality begins to settle in. The adrenaline fades. The visitors become fewer. And that is when it hits: This is real. This is our life now. That moment can be heavy. It can feel lonely, terrifying, or even surreal. But it is also the beginning of something else: the slow, steady process of adjusting. This chapter is about what that process looks like - for your loved one, and for you.

A New Routine, a New Rhythm

Life after spinal injury does not go "back to normal." It becomes a new normal. That means new routines, new challenges, and new ways of doing even the most basic things.

There may be routines for:
- Bowel and bladder care
- Skin checks and pressure relief
- Transferring between bed, chair, toilet, car
- Taking medications
- Using equipment like hoists, wheelchairs, or ventilators
- Scheduling regular physio or care support

At first, these things can feel overwhelming. Even getting out of bed may take time, steps, planning. But I have seen it time and time again - what once seemed impossible becomes second nature. You will build systems, find shortcuts, and make the unfamiliar familiar.

The most important thing is: give yourselves grace. This is a learning curve, not a race.

Shifting Roles and Relationships

Spinal injury does not just change the body, it changes relationships. Partners may become carers. Parents may feel helpless. Siblings might withdraw. Everyone's role shifts.

You may find yourself:
- Making decisions your loved one used to make
- Taking on personal care tasks you never imagined
- Feeling responsible for their physical or emotional wellbeing

These shifts can strain even the strongest relationships. They can bring up guilt, resentment, frustration, and fatigue. That is normal. And it does not mean you are doing anything wrong.

Honest communication is key. So is professional support. You might need family therapy or space to speak to someone outside your circle. That is not failure - it is wisdom.

Letting Go of the Before

Grief is a constant companion after spinal injury - grief for what was lost, for who someone used to be, for the life that once seemed certain. And it is not just the injured person who feels this. Families carry their own kind of grief.

You might grieve:
- The future you imagined
- The ease of spontaneous days
- The freedom from fear or planning
- The roles you each used to play

And yet, here is what I have learned: grief and joy can exist side by side. You do not have to "move on" from what was lost to enjoy what is still here. In fact, that tension - between sadness and gratitude, loss and love - is what makes many post-injury relationships even deeper.

Finding Your Own Balance

One of the biggest dangers for family members is losing themselves in the care role. You may put all your energy into your loved one and leave nothing for yourself.

But here is the truth: You matter too.

You deserve breaks. You deserve emotional support. You deserve joy, hobbies, friendships, laughter and rest.

Creating a sustainable "new normal" means:
- Accepting help from others
- Taking regular time away from the care role
- Saying yes to counselling or therapy for yourself
- Building a support network of people who get it (not just people who mean well)

Reclaiming Joy in New Forms

The "new normal" is not all hospital beds and care routines. There's still room for fun, intimacy, ambition, and adventure. It may look different, but it is still real.

I have seen people go on cruises, fall in love again, go on to have families, become parent, start businesses, write books, take up painting, return to work, or become mentors to others. You do not have to live a small life because of a spinal injury. And neither does your loved one.

But this takes time. And that is okay.

Final Thoughts

Adjusting does not happen overnight. There is no one-size-fits-all form. But with the right mindset, support and information, it does happen.

Some days will be hard. Some will be easier. And every so often, you will look around at your new routines, your new strength and your new kind of joy - and realise that this life, too, is full of meaning.

One of the moments that reminded me of that happened when a long-term client of mine moved out of his mum's house to live independently. I moved with him, of course, and as we settled into this new chapter, one of the first things we started doing was taking his dog for a walk every day. It turned out to be the simplest and most powerful ice breaker. People would stop and chat - other dog walkers, neighbours, even school kids on their way home. Within just a few months, we knew dozens of names and faces. We felt part of the neighbourhood. Known. Seen. That simple act of going out would have incredible effect on my client - but more about it later.

So go out when you can. Say hello. Let people in, even just a little. You never know what kind of community will grow around you - until you give it that first chance to bloom.

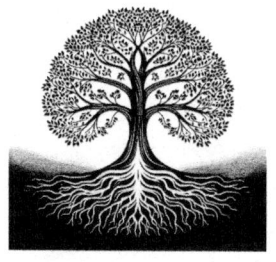

Chapter 4: Understanding Care Needs

Building a Safe, Dignified and Predictable Routine

When a person sustains a spinal cord injury, the body no longer functions in automatic, intuitive ways. This is especially true when it comes to bladder and bowel function. These are not just "personal" matters, they are essential aspects of health, comfort, dignity and independence.

A well managed care routine can mean the difference between stability and crisis, comfort and distress, dignity and distress. In this chapter, we will walk through key areas of spinal care, beginning with one of the most important and often misunderstood: bowel management.

Bowel Management: The Foundation of Stability

For many spinal injury patients, bowel care becomes one of the most essential - and most vulnerable - parts of daily life. After injury, signals between the brain and the bowel are disrupted. This means the bowel no longer empties automatically or in response to brain signals. Without a clear routine, this can lead to:
- Constipation or impaction
- Incontinence
- Autonomic dysreflexia (in high-level injuries)
- Skin damage and infection

The goal is to create a predictable, regular routine that:
- Prevents accidents
- Avoids discomfort
- Reduces health risks
- Offers as much independence, privacy and dignity as possible

Conventional Bowel Care Routine

Many spinal patients follow a structured bowel care routine every day or every other day, although frequency can vary by individual.

Key elements typically include:
- Suppository or mini enema (e.g. Bisacodyl or glycerin)
- Digital stimulation (to prompt reflex emptying)
- Manual evacuation if needed
- All done at the same time of day, ideally after a meal to make use of the gastrocolic reflex

This process is usually done in bed or on a toilet/commode with trained support. It takes time, patience, and respect for the individual's dignity. Remember that safely performed bowel management is essential, ensure that it is performed by trined individual ie district nurse or trained carer. It is not just as easy as inserting suppository. There is a lot to know and pay attention to.

Advanced Bowel Management Options

Some people transition to more advanced or tailored methods as they find what works best for their body, lifestyle and care support.

1. Peristeen / Transanal Irrigation Systems

- A water irrigation system that flushes out the bowel using a small catheter inserted into the rectum
- Can offer greater independence, less time-consuming than traditional bowel care
- Often reduces the chance of accidents or unplanned evacuations
- Can be used every 1- 2 day, typically after breakfast
- Patients often report improved confidence and social freedom

Important Note: Training is essential before starting Peristeen. Not everyone is suitable, it of depends on personal circumstances.

2. Stoma Surgery (Colostomy or Ileostomy)

For some individuals, especially those with severe bowel management challenges or frequent complications, a surgical stoma becomes the most appropriate solution.

- A colostomy creates an opening from the colon to the abdominal wall
- Output is collected in an external bag
- Offers a quicker, more predictable alternative to traditional bowel care
- Especially helpful for people with spastic or unpredictable bowels, or for those who struggle with access, positioning, or distress during care

Stomas are sometimes misunderstood or feared, but for many spinal injury patients, they bring freedom, control, and enormous relief.

Bladder Management: Safety and Dignity

Like the bowel, the bladder is controlled by signals from the spinal cord. Injury disrupts these signals, leading to two major issues:
- Urinary retention (inability to empty the bladder fully)
- Urinary incontinence

Without careful management, bladder issues can lead to:
- Urinary tract infections (UTIs)
- Kidney damage
- Autonomic dysreflexia
- Skin breakdown and discomfort

Bladder care is deeply personal, but also good routine is absolutely essential.

Common Management Methods

Managing the bladder after spinal injury is personal, and what works for one person may not work for another. Below are some of the most common approaches:

1. Intermittent Catheterisation (ISC)
- A clean catheter is inserted into the bladder every 4–6 hours and then removed
- Considered the gold standard for long-term bladder health
- Often used by patients with good hand function, or with assistance
- Lower risk of infection than long-term indwelling catheters

If done with assistance, intermittent catheterisation must be carried out by someone trained in the technique by a qualified healthcare professional, as this is a clinical skill.

2. Indwelling Catheters (Foley)
- A catheter stays in the bladder and drains continuously into a collection bag
- Can be inserted via the urethra or as a suprapubic catheter (a small surgical opening through the abdomen)
- May be more convenient in some cases, especially for those with limited hand function
- Carries a higher long-term risk of infection, bladder stones, and other complications

3. Reflex Voiding with Condom Catheters (for some men)
- Uses a sheath worn over the penis (similar to a condom) attached to a drainage bag
- Suitable only for certain spinal injuries and requires specialist input and careful bladder training
- Works best when reflex voiding is reliable and bladder pressure can be controlled safely

4. Urostomy (Urinary Diversion)
- A surgical procedure where urine is diverted through a stoma into an external bag
- Can be considered in complex cases where catheters lead to repeated infections or severe Autonomic Dysreflexia (AD)
- Though more drastic, it can significantly improve safety, comfort, and quality of life in the right circumstances
- Usually recommended only after all other management options have been explored and discussed with a urologist

Whichever method is used; fluid intake, monitoring, and sterile technique are crucial. Family carers should be trained properly and know signs of UTI or catheter blockage.

Care Is a Routine - Not a Guessing Game

Whether it is bowel care, bladder management, pressure area checks, or transfers, the truth is simple: routine saves lives.

Consistency:
- Prevents medical complications
- Builds confidence and predictability
- Reduces fear and embarrassment
- Preserves dignity

But here is the other truth: routines must also be personalised. What works for one person may not work for another. Finding the right care rhythm takes time, trial, and adjustment. And it must always include the voice and preferences of the person at the centre of it all.

Skin Care and Pressure Area Management

Protecting Skin Is Protecting Life
Skin is often taken for granted - until it becomes fragile. For people with spinal injuries, the risk of pressure sores (also called pressure ulcers) is a constant concern. These injuries can develop quickly, heal slowly, and in some cases, become life-threatening.

A pressure sore starts when the skin is under prolonged pressure - often on bony areas like the:
- Sacrum (base of the spine)
- Heels
- Ankles
- Hips

- Shoulder blades
- Sitting bones

When someone loses sensation, they cannot feel the discomfort, that normally triggers us to shift position. That is why prevention is everything.

Daily Skin Checks

Caregivers must visually inspect the skin - especially pressure points - every single day. This helps catch redness, swelling, or breakdown early.

Pressure Relief Techniques:
- Regular repositioning: Every 2 hours in bed, or per clinical advice (also depending on the mattress)
- Tilt or lift techniques in wheelchairs (manual or power-assisted)
- Specialist mattresses and cushions: Airflow, gel, or memory foam
- Sheepskin or silicone heel protectors and slide sheets to prevent friction

What to Watch For:
- Redness that does not fade after pressure is removed
- Blisters, cracks, or broken skin
- Heat or swelling in high pressure areas
- Fever or fatigue with no clear cause (may indicate infection)

Specialist Support

Many spinal injury patients are under the care of a tissue viability team - nurses trained specifically in skin health and wound care. If pressure damage develops, they should be involved immediately. If your loved one is back at home and there is any concern regarding skin integrity - please do not leave it to "see how it goes", do not wait, call your local district nurses, they will be able to asses if it's something worth worrying about or nothing serious. It is always easier to prevent than heal bad pressure sores, they can appear in a blink of an eye, but healing takes weeks, sometimes even months.

Transfers and Mobility

Freedom Through Safe Movement

Even with limited or no movement below the injury, people with spinal injuries still move - and that movement must be safe, comfortable, and planned.

"Transfers" refer to the process of moving:
- To and from wheelchair
- To and from bed
- To and from toilet, shower chair or commode
- To and from car

Types of Transfers

1. Independent Transfers
- For people with enough upper body strength and balance
- May use a transfer board or sliding board
- Training from an OT or physio is essential for safety

2. **Assisted Transfers**
   - Performed with one or two carers, using manual techniques or a hoist
   - Correct technique is crucial to avoid injury to both patient and carer

3. **Hoist Transfers**
   - Overhead ceiling hoists or mobile floor hoists with slings
   - Provide full support for people with limited mobility
   - Require proper sling fitting and training
   - Used for all major daily transfers when independent movement is not safe

Transfer Training

In rehab, patients often work with physiotherapists and occupational therapists to find the safest and most dignified method for transfers. It is never one-size-fits-all. The goal is always to maximise independence where possible, without compromising safety.

Personal Care and Hygiene

More Than Clean - It is About Dignity

Bathing, brushing teeth, shaving, skincare - these tasks may seem simple, but after spinal injury, they often require support. That does not mean the person has "lost their independence." In fact, they direct their own care even if they need help physically carrying it out.

Bathing and Washing

- Shower chairs, roll-in showers, and shower stretchers make bathing safer
- Some prefer bed baths, especially during illness or fatigue
- Water temperature must be carefully monitored people with SCI may not sense burns
- Make sure skin is throughly dried, pat dry rather than wipe, to prevent skin breakdowns

Oral Care

- Mouth hygiene is crucial for overall health, especially when respiratory issues are present
- Electric toothbrushes can aid those with limited hand function

Grooming and Skin Care

- Daily face and body care helps prevent dryness, rashes, or skin breakdown
- Razor handles, lotion applicators, and long-handled sponges can aid independence

Privacy and Respect

- The person receiving care should always be included in decisions
- Use towels, robes, or positioning to preserve modesty
- Explain each step before and during the process

Caring with someone, not just for them, preserves dignity.

Nutrition and Hydration

Fuel for Healing, Energy, and Health

Good nutrition plays a crucial role in recovery, immune function, and the long-term health of someone with a spinal injury. However, appetite and digestion can change significantly after injury due to:
- Slower bowel motility
- Reduced physical activity
- Medication side effects
- Emotional distress

This makes what, how and when someone eats even more important.

Key Considerations:

- Fibre intake is essential for effective bowel management - too little can cause constipation; too much without water can make it worse.
- Fluids help prevent urinary tract infections, support bowel movement, and keep the skin hydrated. Water is best, but electrolyte drinks can help when needed. And glass of orange juice each day will help with skin integrity and potential healing.
- Balanced meals that include protein, healthy fats, fruits, and vegetables help support wound healing, muscle strength, and energy levels.
- Weight management is important for transfer safety, skin protection, and equipment fitting (e.g. wheelchairs, slings).

Some people may need the support of a dietitian, especially if there are pressure sores, stoma care needs, or diabetes.

Meals are also about pleasure and control, offering choices and involving the person in food planning and cooking can support wellbeing in subtle but powerful ways.

One client I supported had very limited mobility, he could not physically carry out any kitchen tasks on his own. But that never stopped him from being fully involved in every meal. He was with me in the kitchen every day, reading new recipes aloud, guiding me through his old favourites, and making sure everything was just how he liked it. Cooking was not just about food - it was about connection, routine, and joy. He used to joke that between the two of us, we were like Gordon Ramsay - he would do all the swearing, and I would do the cooking. He could not stir the pot himself, but he never missed a chance to be part of what was being made.

Sleep and Positioning

Rest Is not Just Rest - It is Medicine

Sleep can be disrupted after spinal injury for many reasons: pain, spasms, bladder needs, anxiety, or poor positioning. But quality rest is vital for healing, mood, immune strength, and energy.

Key Elements for Quality Sleep:

- Mattresses: Specialist pressure-relieving mattresses (e.g. air flow or alternating pressure systems)

- Pillows and supports: Proper limb positioning to reduce strain, swelling, or nerve pressure
- Repositioning schedules (especially for those with limited mobility): Usually every 2-4 hours, keep in mind that once routine is set and equipment chosen and tested, often repositioning is either less frequent or completely abandoned
- Warmth and temperature: People with SCI often have difficulty regulating body temperature

Sleep routines also matter - creating calm, consistent evenings can reduce anxiety and signal to the body it is time to rest. Some families keep bedside charts to track turning schedules, skin checks, or nighttime catheter drainage.

Emotional Wellbeing Within the Care Routine

Kindness, Control, and the Person Behind the Injury

It is easy to become so focused on tasks: catheterisation, washing, transfers, that we forget care is about people, not just bodies. Every task, no matter how routine, is an opportunity to nurture emotional safety, self-respect, and connection.

Here is how to build that into care:
- Let them direct their care, tell you what to do, in what order, what toiletries to use, which towels they prefer.
- Speak gently and explain: Especially if memory, cognition, or anxiety is involved
- Offer choices: "Would you like to wash your face first or brush your teeth?"

- Involve, do not take over: Let them direct as much of the care as possible if they are not confident enough just yet, to direct the whole routine
- Respect emotions: Some days are harder than others - tears, frustration, and silence are all part of adjusting

It is also okay to laugh. Many spinal injury patients tell me that humour, lightness, and shared jokes are what keep them going. Just because care is serious does not mean it always has to feel solemn.

And finally, care is a two-way street. When possible, carers and family should also look after their own emotional wellbeing. Resentment and burnout are real, and they do not mean you love someone any less - they mean you are human.

In Summary

Understanding care needs is not just about knowing what to do - it is about understanding why it matters, and how to do it well, safely, and compassionately.

When care is consistent, personalised, and respectful, it becomes more than a set of routines - it becomes a foundation of trust, dignity, and wellbeing. And that is what helps people not just survive after spinal injury, but live fully, every day.

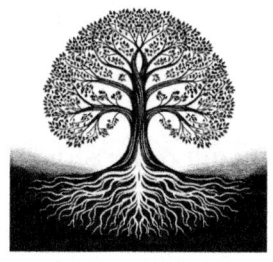

Chapter 5: Choosing and Organising Care

Finding the Right Support for a New Way of Living

One of the most overwhelming realisations for families is this: we cannot do this alone. And you should not have to. Spinal injury care is complex, continuous, and deeply personal. It cannot be handled by one exhausted family member or left entirely to chance.

That is why understanding how to choose, organise, and maintain the right care is one of the most important things you will do - not just for safety, but for dignity, stability, and long-term wellbeing.

Let us walk through what that looks like.

You Do not Have to Be the Carer Alone

Many partners, parents, and children take on care roles out of love - but also because they feel they have to. They may feel pressure to do it all, or guilt if they cannot.

Here is the truth: it is okay to need help. It is okay to ask for help. And it is okay to bring professionals into your home, even if it feels strange at first.

The best care is the kind that is sustainable, safe, and respectful - for both the person receiving care and the one providing it. And that almost always means a team approach.

You Deserve High Quality, Skilled Care

Spinal cord injury brings with it complex clinical needs - not just physical assistance. This is not low level support. Carers must be trained, capable, and confident in the skills required.

You have every right to expect your carers to be:
- Well-trained
- Professional
- Safe
- Respectful
- Competent in clinical tasks
- Attentive to comfort and dignity

And you do not have to settle. I am talking here from my experience, not every care experience is a good one - and I have seen firsthand how damaging poor practice can be, especially when clients do not feel safe enough to speak up.

One client I supported shared some deeply unsettling experiences with an earlier carer. She has arrived hours late, not until the middle of the night - clearly having come straight from a festival or party, in no state to provide safe or respectful care. There was no warning, no apology, and no communication about delays. Her late arrival also meant the outgoing carer could not leave on time, causing even more disruption and stress.
When I asked whether he had reported the behaviour, he told me no - because he was afraid. Afraid that speaking up would get the

carer removed, but that no one would be sent in her place. He did not want to risk being left without support.
We sat down for a long, honest conversation. I reassured him that while that fear is sadly not uncommon, staying silent only enables poor behaviour to continue. If no one holds carers accountable, they are free to carry on acting in ways that are unsafe, unprofessional, and damaging - not just to him, but to others they may support in future.

Advocating for yourself can be difficult, especially when you are already vulnerable. But it is essential. And good care providers will never punish someone for raising a concern - they will see it as a chance to protect others, improve standards, and do the right thing.

That said, I must also add - please be respectful and realistic in your expectations of your carers. Do not insist on unsafe practices and always acknowledge the effort they put into supporting you. Be kind to them. Remember, they need a break too. Many carers are setting aside their own routines, responsibilities, and at times even personal needs to help others live their lives as fully and safely as possible.

Even the most experienced and well trained carer cannot be expected to know your entire routine the moment they walk through the door. If they support multiple clients, each with different preferences, equipment, and ways of doing things, it takes time to adjust. They will learn - it will not take long - but please be patient and understanding when they ask questions or double check how you like something done. Ultimately, this is for your benefit. Good care is personalised, person centred care, and it starts with open, respectful communication.

Types of Care Support

There are several care models depending on your location, funding, and preferences. Each has pros and cons.

1. Family or Informal Care

- Provided by partners, parents, adult children, or friends
- May work well short term or in combination with professional support
- Needs clear boundaries and time for rest
- Should always be paired with proper training from professionals (especially for manual handling, bowel care, catheter care, and pressure care)
- Can be very demanding, leaving no time for any personal time and can be simply draining

2. Live in Carers

- A carer lives in the home and provides full-time support
- Ideal for people with high support needs who want to remain in their own environment
- Can be agency-supplied or employed directly
- Offers continuity and builds strong bonds, but requires mutual trust and personal space

More on Live in Carers – often referred to as Personal Assitants (PAs) or Support Workers (SWs)

They can be:
- Hired directly using Direct Payments or Personal Health Budgets
- Offers flexibility - PAs are chosen and trained based on your needs

- Involves legal responsibilities (contracts, payroll, insurance)

Or:
- Supplied by a care agency who handles recruitment and training
- Can offer security and backup but may lack continuity - depends on an agency
- Quality varies - some agencies provide spinal injury trained specialist carers, they will be trained in bowel care, hoisting and safe moving and handling , ventilators, catheterisation, etc., some may have carers just given basic training - it's important to do your research and ask all the questions - before signing contracts.

3. Domiciliary Care / Visiting Carers

- Carers visit at set times - e.g., morning routines or evening care
- May suit people with partial independence or family support
- Less flexible and may lack continuity
- Rarely you will find here carers trained with clinical skills needed when looking after someone with spinal injury

How to Choose the Right Care

Ask early:

- What level of support is needed 24/7, part-time, or occasional?
- What tasks must carers help with (personal care, transfers, meals, medication)?

- Is the person comfortable with someone living in the home?
- Can the family provide some care and for how long?

Involve your loved one in the decision whenever possible. Even in early stages of injury, having some control over care can help restore dignity.

Pro tip: Some agencies introduce carers before discharge from rehab centre. This allows time for learning the routine and making the home transition smoother.

What to Look for in a Carer

Depending on the injury and care needs, you may require one or two carers at a time, particularly for transfers and any moving handling related tasks.

Carers should be properly trained in:

- Bowel and bladder care (these are clinical tasks)
- Manual handling
- First aid and CPR
- Recognising AD and supporting during episodes of Autonomic Dysreflexia
- Using hoists, slings, and specialist equipment
- Monitoring skin integrity
- Safe handling of medication - if needed
- Delivering safe personal care ie washing/showering, getting client dressed etc

You are fully within your rights to ask for training records or a trial shift. This is your home, your body, your safety.

The Importance of a Good Fit and Continuity

A good carer is worth their weight in gold. The right person becomes more than just help - they become a partner in your daily rhythm. They learn:

- Your preferences
- Early signs of illness or discomfort
- How to communicate with you
- When to step in and when to step back

Continuity matters. High staff turnover creates stress and disrupts routines. Invest time in finding someone who can be a long term part of your support system.

Creating a Healthy Care Dynamic

Care is not just a list of tasks - it is a relationship. And like all relationships, the dynamic between a carer and the person they support must be built on mutual trust, understanding, and respect. When this balance is right, care becomes more than routine - it becomes empowering.

A healthy care relationship should always be grounded in:

- Mutual Respect - Both parties bring value to the relationship. The person receiving care brings knowledge of their own body, needs, and preferences. The carer brings skill, support and a willingness to help. Respect means listening, learning and working together.

- Communication - Open, honest dialogue helps prevent misunderstandings and resentment. Clear communication about needs, routines, boundaries and emotions allows care to be delivered in a way that feels safe and personalised.
- Boundaries - Healthy boundaries protect both the person receiving care and the carer. While care can become close and personal, it is important to remember this is still a professional relationship. Carers are not emotional stand-ins for family, partners, or friends. Kindness and connection are essential, but boundaries ensure that neither party feels pressured, confused, or overwhelmed.
- Dignity - Dignity is at the heart of good care. It means preserving a person's independence wherever possible, respecting their choices and never forgetting their humanity, even in the most intimate or vulnerable moments.

The Person Receiving Care Should:

- Give input on their schedule and preferences - Care should be led by the person wherever possible. When someone is asked how and when they would like something done, it reinforces their autonomy and sense of control.
- Be treated as an equal - Needing support does not mean becoming passive. The person receiving care should always be seen as a partner in the process, not a passive recipient.
- Be addressed directly - Conversations about care should involve the person it concerns. Talking over someone, or about them as if they are not present, undermines their dignity and independence.
- Have privacy, dignity and autonomy protected - Privacy in personal care, choice in daily routines, and the right to make decisions, even imperfect ones, are all essential. Good care uplifts a person's sense of self, rather than replacing or diminishing it.

Medication Support

If your care involves medication, your carer must be trained and competent to support this safely.

They should understand:

- Dosage and timing
- Potential side effects or interactions
- Emergency response protocols
- Hygiene and safe storage
- Record keeping

Even if you usually self manage, your carer should be confident stepping in when needed. Only trained individuals should administer medications or assist with clinical tasks. Support with medication should include record keeping.

A Personal Note from Me, as a Carer

I have worked in this field for nearly two decades, but one of the most meaningful experiences of my life was the 15 years I spent working exclusively with just one client.

When I was first assigned to him, I was told he could be difficult, short tempered, demanding. But I never saw nor experienced that. I saw someone who had been through something life changing and just wanted to be heard. He had routines that worked for him, strong opinions, a sharp wit, and two dogs who were the centre of his world. We clicked quickly. He guided me through his care, and I followed his lead. And once he realised I understood he was in charge he asked me to stay as his regular PA. I gladly did.

Here is the one thing I have learned above all else: communicate.

Even the most experienced carer is walking in blind on the first day. Your voice, your routine, your preferences - that is what shapes good care.

If it is you receiving care, do not be afraid to say (or encourage you loved one to speak up for themselves):

- "I like this towel for my face."
- "I need to be hoisted this way."
- "Please ask before adjusting my chair."

A written plan helps, but nothing replaces person's input. A good carer listens, learns, and respects your way of doing things.

In Summary

Good care is more than keeping someone safe. It is about:

- Dignity
- Choice
- Routine
- Trust
- Connection

Whether you are providing care yourself, hiring professionals, or finding a balance between the two - remember, you do not have to do it all alone. Your role is not to carry everything, but to build a system that truly works for you and your loved one.

Care is never one-size-fits-all. Every situation is unique, and what matters most is creating a supportive structure tailored to your needs. With the right people in place, a clear and realistic plan, and open, ongoing communication, care becomes something empowering - not just for the person receiving it, but for everyone involved. It can bring clarity, confidence, and even a sense of purpose.

And never underestimate the power of a shared laugh. In the midst of challenges, humour can be a remarkable ice breaker - easing tense moments, building connection and making even the most difficult situations feel a little lighter.

With a strong foundation, you are not just managing - you are thriving. And together, you can become unstoppable.

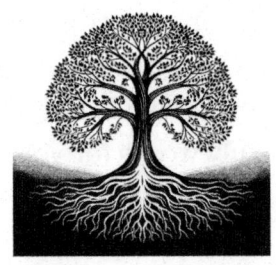

Chapter 6: Coming Home - Adapting Your Home and Building Independence

Leaving hospital or a spinal rehabilitation centre is often a long awaited milestone - but it can also feel daunting. After weeks or months in a specialist setting with trained staff, returning home may raise practical questions, fears, and logistical challenges.

But with the right adaptations and support, home can once again become a space of safety, comfort, and even freedom.

The Transition: From Hospital to Home

Discharge does not mean someone has recovered - it simply means they are ready to continue their journey outside of hospital. This phase is about continuing rehabilitation at home, creating the right environment to live well, and supporting as much independence as possible.

Before discharge, the spinal unit team - usually including an occupational therapist (OT), physiotherapist, social worker, and discharge coordinator - should complete a home assessment and create a discharge plan.

This includes:

- Ensuring essential equipment is in place
- Identifying access barriers (stairs, steps, bathrooms)
- Training for family or carers in manual handling and care routines
- Planning for continued therapy, supplies, and support

Common Home Adaptations

Every home is different, and so are the needs of each person with a spinal injury. However, some common adaptations often include:

Access and Entry
- Ramps or platform lifts for doorways with steps
- Widened doorways for wheelchair access
- Automatic or low threshold doors
- If possible - accessible garden access

Bedroom
- Profiling bed (adjustable height, head/foot elevation)
- Pressure relief mattress
- Ceiling or mobile hoist for transfers if needed
- Room for a carer if needed

Bathroom
- Wet room or level-access shower
- Shower chair/ commode chair, or toilet risers
- Grab rails and non-slip flooring
- Lowered sink and easy tap

Kitchen
- Lowered counters or pull-out shelves
- Side-opening ovens and induction hobs
- Room under sink or counters for wheelchair users

Living Areas
- Furniture rearranged for wheelchair space (including turning point)
- Smooth, hard flooring instead of thick carpets
- Accessible light switches, sockets, and thermostats

Environmental Control Systems (ECS)

Independence at the touch of a button

Environmental Control Systems allow someone with limited mobility to control parts of their home using voice commands, switches, or even eye-gaze systems.

Common ECS functions include:

- Lights, blinds, and heating
- Television, audio, and computer access
- Phone or intercom systems
- Door entry and locks
- Emergency call systems

ECS can be as simple as Alexa or Google Home, or more advanced systems installed via specialist services like Possum or Smartbox. These technologies can transform daily life - giving people control, privacy, and a greater sense of autonomy.

Equipment: What You Might Need

The spinal unit or local community OT will usually help arrange core equipment before discharge. This may include:

- Wheelchair (manual or power)
- Cushions and pressure-relief seating
- Hoists (ceiling or mobile)
- Transfer boards or slide sheets
- Profiling bed and pressure relive mattress
- Shower and commode chairs (often it is 2 in1)

If certain items are not provided by the NHS or social care, they can often be rented, bought second-hand, or funded through charitable grants.

It is important to know not all equipment fits everyone. People vary in size, strength, sensation, injury level, and preferences. The wrong equipment - like an ill-fitting cushion or an oversized shower chair - can cause more harm than good.

That is why staying in contact with your occupational therapist is essential. They can:

- Assess your needs in your own environment
- Recommend the most suitable equipment for safety and comfort
- Arrange adjustments or replacements if something is not working
- Help apply for funding or supplier support if specialist kit is needed

Equipment should support your daily routine - not create new problems. Do not be afraid to ask for changes if something does not feel right. Getting the right fit can make all the difference to comfort, dignity, and independence.

Adapting for the Future, Not Just the Present

Adapting your home after a spinal cord injury is not a one time event, it is an evolving process. Needs change over time. Abilities fluctuate. And what may have seemed unnecessary, out of reach, or even impossible in the early stages of recovery might later become essential or finally achievable. We are not static beings. Our lives shift, and our environments should be able to shift with us. Technology constantly evolves bringing new equipment and solutions.

In the beginning, the focus is often on immediate access and safety - getting through doorways, managing transfers, preventing pressure injuries. But as time goes on, new priorities often emerge: independence, privacy, comfort, control. That is why it is important to revisit your setup regularly and ask, "What would make life easier or more empowering now?"

One of my clients lived for nearly ten years without an environmental control system. He had to rely on others to open windows, unlock doors and let him outside. It chipped away at his independence and left him feeling powerless in his own home. Eventually, his family contacted the local council's home improvement grant team. After an assessment, he was approved for a system that gave him full control over doors and windows, allowing him to let in fresh air, go outside to play with his dog, and come back in without waiting for someone to assist him.

That one change transformed his daily life. He went from waiting to deciding. From being dependent to being in charge.

Adaptations are not just about access - they are about dignity, autonomy, and living on your terms. And sometimes, the right time for a change comes years after the injury. That is perfectly okay.

Maintenance and Servicing of Equipment

Once you are home, it is not just about having the right equipment - it is about keeping it in safe, working condition. Whether your wheelchair, hoist, profiling bed, or pressure relieving mattress was provided by the NHS, a community equipment service, or purchased privately, regular servicing is essential. Servicing equipment regularly must be done, to keep both person and their PA safe.

NHS or local authority provided equipment is usually maintained by a contracted service, keep the contact details easily accessible, and do not hesitate to call if something stops working or becomes unsafe. For privately purchased equipment, it is your responsibility to arrange regular maintenance through the supplier or an approved service provider.

Routine checks can prevent serious incidents.

I once supported a client who had a near miss during a standard bedtime transfer. As we hoisted him onto the bed, I saw the mattress suddenly drop through the frame - panels that should have supported it had collapsed. We quickly transferred him to his shower chair and began checking the frame. It turned out that screws in the adjustable section of the bed had come loose, and the support panels were no longer secured. Thankfully, the second carer was handy with DIY and was able to temporarily stabilise the bed. Equipment services were called the next morning to inspect and reinforce the rest of the frame, ensuring the fault did not reoccur.

That situation could have been much worse. Always report faults promptly, keep track of servicing dates, and never try to 'make do' with damaged or unstable equipment. Your safety depends on it.

Funding and Grants

Adapting a home can be expensive - but there is help available.

Disabled Facilities Grant (DFG – England, Wales, NI)

- Means tested grant for essential home adaptations
- Up to £30,000 (England) / £36,000 (Wales)
- Must apply through your local council
- Usually requires an OT assessment

Scotland: Equipment and Adaptations

- Managed through local health and social care partnerships
- Grants or help-in-kind are available depending on need

Other Potential Sources

- Charities such as The ACT Foundation, Turn2Us, or Independence at Home

- Housing associations may fund adaptations for tenants
- Access to Work (for adaptations related to employment)
- Military charities (for veterans)

Tip: Keep all medical documentation and OT assessments handy - they will be needed for funding applications.

The Emotional Side of Coming Home

Returning home after spinal injury is emotional. Even with the right equipment and changes, it is not "the same" home. It may feel unfamiliar, too small, or filled with memories of "before."

This is normal. Many families report feeling a mix of relief, sadness, fear, and guilt. These feelings often ease with time - and with the development of a new daily rhythm.

Talk about it. Let yourself grieve the changes. But also celebrate the return to your space. Home, once adapted, can be a place of healing, comfort and independence once more.

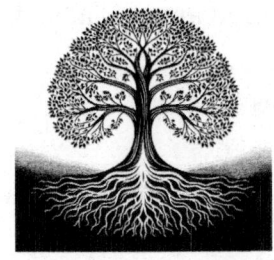

Chapter 7: Daily Routines and Rebuilding Confidence at Home

Finding Normality in the Everyday

After a spinal injury, the hospital days are structured - nurses on schedule, rehab sessions booked, meals served. But once you're home, structure often falls away. The days can start to blur, confidence can wobble, and families may feel unsure how to keep things moving forward.

This chapter is about reclaiming rhythm. It is about showing that daily life, though different, can still be meaningful, satisfying, and full of small victories.

Why Routine Matters

For people with spinal cord injury (SCI), a well structured routine is not just convenient, it is essential.

It helps with:

- Bladder and bowel management (timing is key to avoiding accidents)
- Pressure care (regular repositioning and skin checks)
- Energy levels and fatigue management

- Mental health, reducing anxiety and giving the day shape
- Maintaining independence by repeating and refining tasks

But it is also about restoring normality. A routine reminds someone that their life has not disappeared, it is just being rebuilt, one piece at a time.

Creating a Personalised Daily Routine

Each person's injury is different. So is each home. So is each family. But a basic routine often includes:

- Morning care (washing, dressing, bladder routine, bowel care if scheduled)
- Meals (including time for meal prep or carer support)
- Exercise/physiotherapy (stretching, standing frame, movement)
- Rest periods (fatigue is common)
- Repositioning or transfers (based on pressure care plan)
- Hobbies or mental stimulation (reading, TV, games, creative activities)
- Evening care (catheter checks, medication, wind down routine)

Some people use whiteboards or care logs to track these - especially when working with multiple carers.

Tip: Leave space for flexibility. Routine should support, not control. Life still needs room for spontaneity.

Doing Things for Yourself - Even in Small Ways

Regaining independence can be slow - but incredibly powerful. Even the smallest tasks can build confidence:

- Brushing teeth from bed
- Applying face cream with adaptive aids
- Using voice controls to turn on music or open blinds
- Choosing your own clothes, even if someone else helps dress you
- Making a simple snack or drink using adaptive kitchen tools

These small choices help restore a sense of dignity. They are a quiet but powerful reminder: "This is still my life and I'm still in charge of it." And yes, a lot of those will dependant on level of injury, and regained abilities or equipment available - but it is important to aim for those moments and to celebrate them!

Encourage involvement in care, not just passivity. Carers should support independence, not replace it. It may be easier and quicker to have something done by the carer, but it is so much more satisfying to see person doing it themselves. Especially for them. It builds their confidence and believe in their own abilities.

Confidence Is Rebuilt in Layers

Confidence does not come back all at once. It grows slowly.

One of my clients once said, "The first time I brushed my own hair again, I cried. Not because it looked great, but because it was me doing it."

That is what this chapter is about. Those moments.

Confidence grows when:
- A task gets easier
- A carer steps back slightly and it goes fine
- A mishap happens - but it's handled
- A trip out goes well
- Someone realises they can still make choices, still have opinions, still matter

Supporting the Whole Household

Daily routines work best when the whole household understands and supports them. That might mean:
- Ensuring that people involved as all on the same page, know the routine, know their role
- Discussing needs and preferences regularly
- Agreeing quiet times, privacy, or rest periods
- Involving children or partners in a respectful, appropriate way

Family members should not feel like they are in a care unit - but routines help avoid confusion, frustration, and missed steps.

Setting Goals and Continuing Rehabilitation at Home

Rehabilitation does not end when a person leaves hospital, in many ways, it is only the beginning. The home becomes the new setting for rebuilding strength, confidence, and independence. Setting realistic, meaningful goals can help structure daily routines and provide a sense of progress, no matter how small the steps may seem.

Goals do not need to be dramatic or complex. They can be as simple as managing a full morning routine independently, sitting out in the garden each day, preparing a basic meal, or practising transfers from bed to wheelchair with fewer prompts. What matters is that they are personal, achievable and aligned with the person's current ability and long-term hopes.

Continued rehabilitation may involve home visits from physiotherapists or occupational therapists, but just as often, it takes the form of everyday repetition: doing stretches each morning, using assistive equipment correctly, or practising a skill again and again. Progress can be slow - and that is okay. Celebrate small victories. Keep a record of improvements. Even on difficult days, these small efforts are quietly building resilience, strength and confidence.

One of my clients is a perfect example of how consistent effort at home can lead to remarkable progress over time. When I first began supporting him, he used his standing frame two to three times a week. As we settled into a regular routine, he committed to using it daily, gradually building strength and learning how to support himself using his core and abdominal muscles instead of relying heavily on his shoulders for balance. Over two years, his posture improved significantly. There were times when he felt as though he was standing still, making no progress, but I would remind him of how far he had come. In the beginning, he needed a binder every time due to limited control over his diaphragm and breathing, and he would often become lightheaded. Two years later, he was confidently using the standing frame for twice as long, without a binder, and with much more independence.

These are the kinds of gains that can go unnoticed unless we take the time to reflect. They are proof that progress is not always loud or fast, but steady, quiet, and powerful.

Tracking Progress - Not Perfection

If you or your loved one is on this journey, consider keeping a simple record of achievements - no matter how small they may seem. Noting down moments of progress, new skills, or even the return of everyday routines can help shift focus from what has been lost to what is being rebuilt. On the hard days, looking back at how far you have come can offer strength, perspective and hope. Rehabilitation is not a straight line, and it is easy to overlook growth when you are living it day by day, but every effort counts and every step forward matters.

Keep a small journal, logbook, or even a whiteboard of wins:
- "Managed hair care independently today"
- "No help needed for transfer!"
- "Spoke up and changed part of the care routine"
- "Felt stronger after physio"

These are not just notes. They are evidence of growth. They show the person and the family, just how far they have come. Remember: no progress is too small to be proud of.

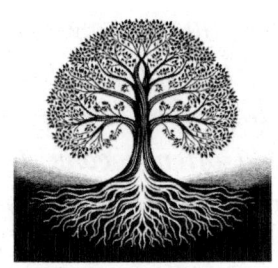

Chapter 8: Risks and How to Manage Them

What to Watch for and How to Stay One Step Ahead

Spinal cord injury does not just affect movement and sensation, it changes how the body functions in nearly every system. This means there are some very medical risks that families need to understand and actively manage.

But here is the key: being aware of these risks does not mean living in fear. It means being prepared. Most of the complications listed here can be managed - or even prevented, if caught early and handled correctly.

Let us walk through them together.

1. Pressure Sores (Pressure Ulcers)

Skin Can Break Down Quickly Without Warning

What it is: A pressure sore is an injury to the skin and underlying tissue caused by prolonged pressure, often over bony areas like the hips, heels, ankles, sacrum, and shoulder blades.

Why it matters: Left untreated, pressure sores can become infected, deepen into muscle or bone, and even become life threatening.

What to look for:
- Redness that does not fade
- Swelling, heat, or pain
- Cracks or open wounds
- Unusual smells or discharge

How to prevent it:
- Daily skin checks - especially on high risk areas
- Use of pressure relieving cushions and mattresses
- Right equipment (OT will help assess for the most fitting equipment and aids)
- Regular repositioning, even in wheelchairs - even a little stretch will help as any movement will change the pressure points.
- Maintaining skin hygiene and good nutrition
- Immediate call to district nurses if any signs appear, they can assess and treat or if they are concerned, they will contact tissue viability team

2. Autonomic Dysreflexia (AD)

A Life-Threatening Emergency That Demands Fast Action

What it is:
Autonomic Dysreflexia (AD) is a sudden, dangerous spike in blood pressure caused by a noxious (irritating or painful) stimulus below the level of spinal injury. It typically affects individuals with injuries at or above T6, and occurs because the brain cannot communicate with the body in the usual way.

When something goes wrong below the injury - like a blocked catheter or full bowel—the body tries to alert you by raising blood pressure. But because the signal cannot reach the brain clearly, the response becomes uncontrolled. Blood vessels constrict, but they do not relax again. Blood pressure continues to climb, and if not treated quickly, AD can lead to stroke, seizure, or cardiac arrest.

To put it simply: if the body detects a problem it cannot process normally, it sounds the alarm through blood pressure. That is why something as small as a twisted leg bag or tight waistband can become a serious emergency for someone with a spinal cord injury.

In general, people with spinal injuries often have low baseline blood pressure. Over time in rehab or at home, you will learn what is "normal" for your loved one - and what an episode of AD feels like. Remember: for someone with SCI, a blood pressure of 130/110 or 145/115 can be life-threatening, even if it would not be alarming in someone else.

Because of this, AD is now treated as a medical emergency, on par with heart attacks and strokes. It must never be ignored.

Common Triggers of AD

- A full bladder (e.g., blocked catheter or overfilled drainage bag)
- Constipation or bowel impaction
- Urinary tract infection (UTI)
- Tight clothing, belts, or abdominal binders
- Pressure on the skin (e.g., from sitting unevenly or creased clothing)

- Ingrown toenails, burns, pressure sores, or even minor injuries
- Sexual stimulation or menstruation

Symptoms to Watch For

- Sudden, severe, pounding headache
- Flushed or red skin above the level of injury (often face and neck)
- Profuse sweating above the injury
- Goosebumps or cold, clammy skin below the injury
- Nasal congestion
- Anxiety or a feeling of doom
- Slow or irregular pulse (though it may also rise in some cases)
- Blurred vision, dizziness, or nausea

Each person will have their own pattern of symptoms - learn them, and do not rely only on textbook signs. The person experiencing AD may not always notice the early signs themselves, so it is important that carers, family members and PAs remain alert.

Real Life Example: The Unexpected Trigger

I once supported a client who began showing all the signs of AD - headache, rising blood pressure, flushed skin - but we could not find the cause. We checked everything: catheter, clothing, pressure areas, bowel routine. Still, his blood pressure kept rising, and we were about to call 999 when, quite unexpectedly, he passed wind. Within a minute, his blood pressure dropped, and he started to feel better. Moments later, he was back to normal.

What triggered his AD? Trapped wind. Something that would be insignificant for most people had put him at real risk. That moment stayed with me - it is why I always say: do not underestimate AD, and do not delay. If you see symptoms, act. Even small things can have a big impact.

Immediate Steps to Take

1. Sit the person upright
This is usually the first step, as it helps lower blood pressure by encouraging blood to pool in the lower body. However, positioning can vary depending on individual needs or medical advice. Make sure that everyone involved in care is familiar with the specific positioning recommended for your loved one. This should be clearly recorded in both their everyday care plan and hospitalisation plan (we will talk more about that later), so there is no confusion in an emergency.

2. Loosen tight clothing or accessories.
Belts, waistbands, abdominal binders, or tight shoes may be causing pressure.

3. Check the bladder.
- Drain the catheter bag.
- Look for kinks or blockages.
- If trained, flush or change the catheter.
- If not trained or unsure, call for emergency medical support (district nurse or 999 if needed)

4. Check the bowel.
- If bowel care is due and you are trained, perform it immediately.
- If not, remove any obvious triggers and monitor closely.

5. Remove other potential triggers.
- Check for skin issues, ingrown toenails, pressure spots, or hidden injuries.

6. If symptoms persist or the cause is unclear: Call 999.
Let them know the person has a spinal cord injury and is experiencing Autonomic Dysreflexia. Paramedics should treat it as seriously as a stroke or heart attack.

When to Call 999 Immediately

- If symptoms do not improve after initial steps
- If the cause is unclear
- If the person is showing signs of severe distress (e.g., chest pain, visual changes, confusion)
- If this is their first episode of AD
- If you are not trained to resolve the trigger

Medication for Autonomic Dysreflexia

Most people with SCI, who are at risk of AD, will be prescribed emergency medications to lower blood pressure rapidly. These should be used only in emergency and as prescribed.

Common options include:
- Nifedipine (Adalat): Fast-acting capsule placed under the tongue
- GTN spray: Used to lower BP quickly, spray in person's mouth, under their tongue

Medication should always be recorded in the care plan, and emergency services should be informed about name of the medication, dose and amount administered.

Every Person Should Have an AD Response Plan

Work with your spinal injury specialist or rehabilitation team to create a personalised AD response plan, including:

- Usual blood pressure range
- Known triggers and typical symptoms
- Step-by-step actions
- Emergency medication instructions
- When to call 999

This protocol should be:
- Kept at home in the care folder
- Shared with all carers and family
- Included in hospital and emergency files
- Stored in a wallet card or phone app if out in public

Training and Preparedness

Anyone involved in care must be trained to:
- Recognise symptoms of AD
- Respond confidently and quickly
- Know when and how to give medication
- Know when to escalate and call 999

Many spinal rehab units provide emergency AD cards. Keep one in the wallet, next to the bed, or in a wheelchair pouch.

The Importance of Record Keeping

When it comes to Autonomic Dysreflexia, keeping a detailed record of each episode is not just helpful - it can be essential. AD can be life-threatening if not recognised and treated promptly and knowing your personal triggers plays a vital role in prevention. Recording each incident - including the date, time, suspected or confirmed trigger, symptoms, and how it was managed - can help identify patterns over time. This allows both the person affected and the care team to anticipate and reduce future risks more effectively.

Beyond the clinical benefits, accurate documentation can also support care funding reviews. Records of AD episodes clearly demonstrate the complexity and seriousness of the person's health needs. They show how essential timely and skilled care is in maintaining safety and wellbeing, how dangerous it could be for the person to be without proper support.

Most professional care agencies will be required to record each instance of AD as a formal incident due to its medical severity. However, it is also a good idea for individuals and families to keep their own log. This extra layer of documentation can be particularly helpful in reviews, appeals, or when transitioning between services, making sure that no detail is missed and that the reality of day-to-day risk management is fully understood by all involved.

Final Word on AD

Autonomic Dysreflexia is serious - but with knowledge, training and fast response, it is entirely manageable. Lives have been saved by early action. Knowing the signs, responding with calm urgency, and trusting your instincts can make all the difference.

And sometimes, yes - something as small as trapped wind can be the cause. That is why we check everything. That is why we act without delay. Because with AD, every second counts.

3. Urinary Tract Infections (UTIs)

Common, But Not to Be Ignored

What it is: An infection anywhere in the urinary system, often caused by bacteria introduced through catheter use or incomplete emptying of the bladder.

Signs to watch for:
- Cloudy or strong-smelling urine
- Increased spasms
- Fever or chills
- Lethargy or sudden confusion (especially in older adults)
- Autonomic dysreflexia symptoms

Prevention tips:
- Practice clean or sterile catheter care technique (always wear gloves to empty or change catheter bag etc)
- Encourage regular fluid intake
- Monitor urine colour and output daily

Bladder health is a lifelong priority after SCI. UTIs are common, but preventable with vigilance and good technique.

4. Constipation and Bowel Complications

Unpredictable Bowels Can Lead to Serious Discomfort

As discussed in Chapter 4, bowel management is a vital part of health after spinal injury.

A missed routine or poor diet can cause:
- Constipation
- Bowel impaction
- Incontinence
- Autonomic dysreflexia

Warning signs:
- No bowel movement in several days
- Distended abdomen
- Nausea or loss of appetite
- Accidents outside of routine
- Fatigue or confusion

Prevention:
- Stick to the bowel care schedule religiously
- Balance fibre and water intake
- Use prescribed methods (suppositories, irrigation, etc.) correctly
- Seek medical advice early if something feels "off"

Never underestimate the power of a well maintained bowel routine. It is one of the most effective ways to protect dignity and comfort.

5. Respiratory Infections

Especially Risky in High Level Injury

Spinal cord injuries, especially those at the cervical (neck) level, can significantly impact respiratory function. This is because the muscles involved in breathing - including the diaphragm, intercostal muscles, and abdominal muscles - may be weakened or completely paralysed depending on the level and severity of the injury.

One of the biggest challenges is the reduced ability to cough effectively. Coughing is essential for clearing mucus and secretions from the lungs. When this function is impaired, mucus can build up, increasing the risk of:
- Chest infections
- Pneumonia
- Atelectasis (partial or complete lung collapse due to mucus obstruction)

Even something as minor as a common cold can quickly develop into a more serious respiratory condition, so proactive care is essential.

Prevention and Support Strategies:

- Regular chest physiotherapy and assisted coughing help move and clear mucus from the lungs. This might involve manual techniques or caregiver support. (Assisted coughing involves applying pressure to the abdomen or chest during an exhale to help push air out more forcefully, mimicking a natural cough – anyone can be trained to do this by respiratory physiotherapist)

- Cough assist machines or suction equipment can be used when the individual is unable to generate a strong enough cough on their own.
- Breathing exercises and use of devices like incentive spirometers encourage deeper breaths and help keep the lungs expanded.
- Avoiding exposure to illness is crucial. This includes staying away from anyone ill and managing cold or flu symptoms as soon as they arise.
- Vaccinations - such as the annual flu jab and pneumonia vaccine - are strongly recommended to reduce the risk of serious respiratory complications.

For individuals with high-level injuries, respiratory support may be an ongoing part of daily care. Understanding the early signs of respiratory decline and having a clear action plan in place can make a crucial difference in preventing emergencies.

6. Spasms and Pain

Sometimes Functional, Sometimes Distressing

Spasticity - meaning involuntary muscle spasms or stiffness - is a common result of spinal cord injury (SCI), particularly in individuals with incomplete injuries or upper motor neuron involvement. These spasms can range from mild twitching to strong, painful contractions that affect large muscle groups.

Spasticity can cause:
- Pain or discomfort
- Disrupted sleep

- Increased difficulty with transfers, dressing, or personal care
- Sudden, uncontrolled movement, which can sometimes be unsafe

However, not all spasticity is negative. In some cases, it can provide functional benefits - for example, helping with standing or maintaining posture. Each person's experience with spasticity is different, and management often involves finding the right balance between reducing discomfort and preserving any useful tone or movement.

Neuropathic pain is another frequent and often misunderstood challenge. Unlike muscular or joint pain, this type of pain stems from damage to the spinal cord or nerves. It is often described as:
- Burning
- Stabbing
- Tingling
- Electric shock-like

What makes neuropathic pain especially difficult is that it may occur in areas that no longer have normal sensation. It can be unpredictable, fluctuating in intensity, and triggered by temperature changes, movement, stress, or seemingly nothing at all.

One of my clients suffered from severe neuropathic pain that would flare up every time he transferred onto the bed. For the next hour or two, he would scream in pain and sweat profusely, completely overwhelmed by the intensity of the sensation. It was heartbreaking to witness, especially as no one could pinpoint the exact cause - or offer effective relief. Only after lying still for a prolonged period, once his body finally relaxed, would the pain slowly fade away. It was a stark reminder that not all pain has a visible trigger or easy solution.

Management Strategies Include:

- Medication - Such as Baclofen (for spasticity) and Gabapentin or Pregabalin (for nerve pain). Finding the right combination often takes time and close monitoring.
- Physiotherapy and stretching - Can ease stiffness, manage spasms, and promote comfort.
- Advanced therapies - Options like Botox injections, nerve blocks, or intrathecal baclofen pumps may be offered in severe cases.
- Keeping a pain diary - Helps track patterns, identify potential triggers, and guide treatment adjustments.

Spasms and pain - especially when persistent and unexplained - can take a heavy toll on both the individual and those supporting them. Compassion, patience, and a personalised approach are essential to improving comfort and preserving dignity.

7. Mental Health Strain

Do not Overlook the Invisible Risks

Spinal cord injury affects far more than the body. It brings an immense emotional and psychological toll - not only for the person who has been injured but also for their loved ones. Depression, anxiety, grief, and post traumatic stress are common and very real responses to such a life altering event. Everything changes - daily routines, independence, identity, future plans, and social roles. And with those changes come waves of loss, uncertainty, and adjustment that take time and care to process.

From my experience, many people with spinal cord injuries go through periods of deep emotional struggle. Depression is particularly common. It can creep in quietly or hit all at once, and sometimes, it is hidden behind frustration, anger, or withdrawal. It is important to understand that this response is not a weakness - it is a natural reaction to trauma and drastic change.

One of my clients sadly struggled with depression. There were times he truly felt that his life was worthless. His behaviour changed dramatically - he would swing between being silent and withdrawn, and suddenly lashing out, saying deeply hurtful things to those closest to him. He stopped eating properly, lost a significant amount of weight, and seemed to be fading before our eyes. It was not until his brother and sister in law sat him down and had a raw, honest conversation, telling him how painful it was to watch him hurt and neglect himself, and how even his beloved nieces had noticed that their fun, playful uncle was no longer there, that something shifted. That moment, painful but rooted in love, was the catalyst for him seeking help. It showed me just how powerful honest conversations can be. Even difficult truths, when spoken from a place of care, can spark real change.

Sometimes things will get hard, difficult, messy and heavy. Mental health struggles do not come with a warning, and none of us are immune. One of the most valuable lessons I have learned is that when things are tough, the best you can do is to take each day as it comes.

During one particularly challenging time, client of mine experienced a significant decline in mental health. Each day brought new uncertainty - emotionally, behaviourally and practically. It was hard on me, but it was so much harder on him. I made a decision that carried me through: at the end of each day, I let that day go. No dwelling, no resentment, no carrying forward the weight of what was said or done in distress.

He would often ask me at bedtime, "Was I awful today? Are you upset with me?" And even on the hardest days, I would say "No, we are good." Not because everything had been easy, but because I knew he was already burdened by his illness. Adding guilt or shame would serve no one. Every morning was a clean slate. I highly recommend this to anyone supporting someone through emotional struggle.

There will be days when the weight of the injury becomes overwhelming and your loved one may lash out or retreat. Do not take it personally. Address it, yes, but let it go. Do it for them and do it for yourself. Holding on to every hard moment only makes the load heavier.

Signs to Look For:
- Withdrawal or becoming unusually quiet
- Tearfulness, irritability, or mood swings
- Changes in sleep or appetite
- Feelings of hopelessness, worthlessness, or loss of interest in previously enjoyed activities

Mental health struggles are not always obvious. Sometimes they show up in silence, sarcasm, or exhaustion. If something feels off, it is worth talking about, even if it is uncomfortable.

What Helps:
- Counselling or therapy - Especially with professionals who understand disability, grief, or trauma. Therapy is not just about "fixing" something; it is a space to explore, process, and regain control.
- Peer support groups - Many spinal centres and charities offer these, and hearing from others who have been through it can be incredibly validating and uplifting.
- Open conversations with family and friends - Creating a safe space where feelings can be expressed without pressure or judgment can foster connection and prevent isolation.
- Medication - If appropriate, can help manage symptoms, and should never be seen as shameful or a sign of failure.

Families Need Support Too

Carers often carry an enormous emotional load. It is not uncommon to push your own feelings aside while focusing on the needs of the person you love. But your wellbeing matters just as much. You cannot pour from an empty cup. Talking to someone - a friend, counsellor, peer - can offer perspective and relief. You deserve support, too.

Please do not ignore the signs. Whether you are the person with the injury or someone who loves and supports them, seeking help is an act of strength - not weakness. With the right support, people do find their way through the darkness. They rebuild. They adapt. And they reconnect with joy, even if it looks different than before.

8. Temperature Dysregulation

The Body Does not Always Know Hot from Cold

One lesser-known but serious risk after spinal injury, especially injuries at or above T6, the body can lose its ability to automatically regulate temperature. The brain's signals to sweat, constrict blood vessels, or adjust circulation may not reach below the level of injury. To put it simply the brain's communication with the parts of the body responsible for heating and cooling is disrupted. That means the body does not regulate temperature in the usual way - it adapts as best it can. Often adapting to the temperature around it. The body does not actively maintain balance. Instead, it becomes more passive and reactive, which means a person can quickly become too hot or too cold without the typical warning signs or physical responses like sweating or shivering.

What does that mean?
- The person may not sweat normally below the injury level (or at all)
- They may become dangerously hot without noticing it
- Or struggle to stay warm, even in moderate temperatures
- External signs may not match internal body temperature

Risks include:
- Heatstroke in warm weather or hot environments
- Hypothermia in cooler weather or after bathing
- Fatigue, confusion, headaches, and dizziness due to overheating

- Skin damage from external heat sources (e.g., hot water bottles, electric blankets)

How to manage it:
- Monitor room temperature carefully - avoid extremes
- Use fans, cooling vests, or misting sprays during hot weather
- Stay out of direct sunlight for long periods, especially in summer
- Avoid tight or insulating clothing that traps heat – dress for the weather
- Encourage fluid intake to support natural cooling
- In cold weather, layer clothing and use blankets - but avoid direct heat against skin that lacks sensation
- Do not rely on sweating or shivering as a signal - go by the environment and routine checks

Carers and family must stay vigilant, especially during weather changes, long car journeys, or holidays abroad. Temperature regulation is not just a comfort issue - it can become a life-threatening situation if not taken seriously.

- Avoid prolonged exposure to direct sunlight, especially during hot summer days.
- Limit time spent in direct sun, particularly in warm weather, to prevent overheating.
- Try to stay in shaded or cool areas during summer, as direct sunlight can quickly lead to overheating.

9. Hospitalisation Care Plan Matters

If the worst happens and your loved one needs to be admitted to hospital, preparation is key. Hospital environments are not always equipped to meet the complex needs of someone with a spinal cord injury, especially when it comes to skin care, bowel routines, transfers, or recognising signs of Autonomic Dysreflexia. Having a clear, well documented hospital plan can make all the difference - ensuring your loved one receives the right care, and that their voice, needs, and safety are not lost in the chaos of an unfamiliar setting.

For anyone living with a spinal cord injury, having a hospitalisation care plan ready and up to date can make a huge difference in a medical emergency or planned admission. Unlike a general care plan, this is a more focused, easy to follow document designed specifically for healthcare teams unfamiliar with the person's daily needs. Hospitals can be overwhelming, especially when clinical staff are not trained in spinal injury care. A well prepared hospitalisation plan bridges that gap - it gives nurses and doctors a clear picture of who the patient is, what risks they face, and what is needed to keep them safe and comfortable.

A good plan should include: the person's name, how they prefer to be addressed, contact details for next of kin, carer, and care manager (if using an agency), key contacts like district nurses, and a brief medical history highlighting any pressure sores, spinal level, and known risks. It should include detailed guidance on Autonomic Dysreflexia (AD) - what their individual triggers are, how it presents in their body, and exactly how to relieve it. It should also include their bowel and bladder routines, skin care requirements, equipment they rely on (such as a pressure-relieving mattress), a full medication list, and clear notes on who provides which aspects of care (and whether a carer will remain in hospital with them).

Having this plan on hand avoids dangerous delays, reduces repeated explanations, and ensures that the care delivered in hospital stays consistent with what is needed at home. It is something that should be reviewed and updated regularly, especially after any change in routine or medical status. In urgent moments, this simple document becomes a lifeline - not just for the person with the injury, but for every healthcare professional trying to support them.

Advocacy in Hospital: Why Your Voice Matters

Even with a well documented care plan, advocacy remains essential. Hospital staff are often highly skilled in responding to the medical emergency that brought your loved one in, but that does not always mean they understand the unique needs of someone living with a spinal cord injury. Your presence, knowledge and assertiveness can bridge that gap and prevent serious complications.

I have witnessed this firsthand.

One of my clients, while on a hospital ward, was asked by a nurse to "move his legs over." When he explained he was unable to, the nurse responded, "Are you sure?" - a stark reminder of how unaware some staff may be about the realities of spinal cord injury.

In another case, one of my clients began experiencing Autonomic Dysreflexia while admitted to hospital. His hospital plan clearly outlined the risks and protocol for managing AD. I immediately alerted the staff, and though they took his blood pressure, they told me it was "only 150/110" - not recognising that for someone whose usual BP is around 95/75, this was already a warning sign. I explained the situation clearly, but was told someone would return in ten minutes. No one came. My client became increasingly incoherent. I returned to the nurses' station and, quite firmly, some might say rudely, asked the sister in charge, "What are you waiting for? For him to have a stroke, a heart attack, or just die?" That finally got their attention. At this point his BP had risen to over 200. What followed was a rush to stabilise him and manage the cause of AD: multiple doses of Nifedipine and GTN spray, an emergency ICU admission and hours of careful monitoring. It was a terrifying situation and it could have been prevented.

After discharge, my client contacted the hospital's patient advocacy service to raise concerns about the lack of awareness and response. As a result, he was invited to deliver training sessions for nurses and healthcare assistants at that same hospital. Many of them said it was eye opening to hear directly from someone with a spinal injury, to understand what hospital care feels like from the inside.

Never underestimate the power of speaking up. Whether you are a family member, a friend, or a professional carer - your voice may be the one that protects your loved one in a system that is not always built for their needs. Know the care plan. Know the signs. And be ready to act if necessary. Advocacy saves lives.

What to Include in a Hospitalisation Care Plan

- Full name and preferred name or form of address
- Date of birth
- Spinal cord injury level and brief medical background
- Next of kin and emergency contact details
- Current carers' names and contact info (including who provides what support)
- Care manager or agency contact (if applicable)
- District nurse contact details (if involved in care)
- Pressure sore history – current risks or areas of concern
- Details on Autonomic Dysreflexia (AD):
  - Known triggers
  - Typical symptoms
  - Immediate actions to take
  - Prescribed AD medication and where it is kept
- Bladder management routine:
  - Type of catheter used (if any)
  - Frequency of catheterisation
  - Who performs the task (self or carer)
- Bowel management routine:
  - Frequency and method (e.g., digital stimulation, Peristeen, suppositories)
  - Who performs the task
- Skin care needs:
  - Daily checks
  - Moisturisers or creams used
  - Known pressure points or vulnerabilities
- Mobility and transfer needs:
  - Hoisting, slide board, or manual transfers
  - Preferred techniques or equipment

- Specialist equipment needed:
    - Pressure-relieving mattress
    - Wheelchair type and functions
    - Shower chair, standing frame, etc.
- Medication list:
    - Current medications, dosages, and timing
    - Allergy information
- Feeding and nutrition:
    - Special dietary needs or feeding support
- Communication preferences (verbal, non-verbal, use of assistive tech)
- Consent regarding carers in hospital:
    - Will the carer stay with them?
    - Are they authorised to assist with or perform care tasks?

In Summary

Spinal injury carries risks. That is the truth. But risks are not the enemy, being unprepared is. Every risk outlined here can be managed, prevented, or caught early when you know what to look for. Knowledge is power. Routine is protection. And community is support.

With awareness, planning, and the right care in place, spinal injury does not have to mean constant crisis. It can mean stability, confidence, and control.

Below is an example of an action plan for managing Autonomic Dysreflexia (AD). It can be included in a care plan, hospital care plan, or kept easily accessible so carers can act quickly and confidently when needed.

Autonomic Dysreflexia (AD) Emergency Protocol

To be kept with care records, in hospital care plan, and shared with all caregivers.

Name: _____
Date of Birth: _____
Level of Injury: _____
My Usual Blood Pressure is _____
Known to Experience AD: Yes / No
Typical AD Triggers for Me:
- Full bladder / catheter issues
- Bowel-related (constipation, impaction)
- Tight clothing or equipment
- Skin pressure or sore
- Infection (e.g. UTI)
- Other: _____

My Early Warning Signs of AD:
(Check or write in as needed)
- Headache (describe): _____
- Sweating (location): _____
- Facial flushing
- Goosebumps
- Anxiety or unease
- Vision changes
- Other: _____

Immediate Steps:

1. Sit me upright (or you can add position that is best for you in case of AD)

Help me into an upright seated position to lower blood pressure.

2. Loosen anything tight.
Remove belts, abdominal binders, tight socks, shoes, etc.
3. Check for and address common triggers:
- Bladder:
    - Drain catheter
    - Check tubing for blockages or kinks
    - If trained, flush or replace catheter if blocked
- Bowel:
    - Perform bowel routine only if trained and if this is a known cause
    - Do not perform without gloves/lubricant or proper equipment
- Skin:
    - Check for signs of pressure or injury (heels, sacrum, toes, etc.)

Emergency Medication (if prescribed):
- Medication Name: _____
- Dosage/Form: _____
- How to Administer: _____
- Stored: _____
- Only to be used under specific conditions: _____

When to Call 999:
- If symptoms do not resolve quickly after removing the trigger
- If you are unsure of the cause
- If the person becomes unresponsive, dizzy, or severely distressed
- If blood pressure remains dangerously high

When calling:
State: "This person has a spinal cord injury and is experiencing

autonomic dysreflexia. This is a life-threatening emergency that requires immediate medical attention."
Spinal Centre / Consultant Contact:
Name: _____
Phone: _____
Hospital: _____

Emergency Notes / Additional Instructions:

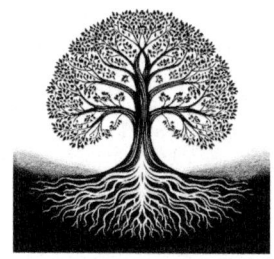

Chapter 9: Learning, Purpose, and Returning to Work

Education, Employment, and Redefining What Is Possible

After a spinal cord injury, it can feel as though many doors suddenly close. A loved one may have had to leave a job they were passionate about. Their education may have been interrupted, or their plans for the future may now feel uncertain. For families, it is heartbreaking to watch someone they care about question their purpose or identity.

But the journey does not end here. Life can still hold opportunities for learning, growth, and contribution. Whether through work, study, volunteering, or creative expression, many people with spinal injuries go on to rediscover, or redefine, their sense of purpose. And with the right support, it is entirely possible.

Finding something meaningful to engage in is not just about income or routine. It supports mental wellbeing, confidence, and connection. It helps to rebuild identity and pride. That matters, not just for the person with the injury, but for the entire family.

Education After Spinal Injury

Regardless of whether someone left school early, was in the middle of a degree, or never had the opportunity to study before, education remains a valid and valuable option after a spinal injury – and yes, I did work with a client who was in full time education studying at university, living in a student accommodation along with his carer.

People can now study:
- From home through online or distance learning
- At their own pace with part time or flexible options
- With physical, sensory, or learning support in place

Colleges, universities, and adult learning centres are legally required to make reasonable adjustments for disabled students. These can include:
- Step free access and mobility support
- Assistive technology and note taking support
- Extra time for coursework or exams
- Flexibility around attendance or deadlines

The Disabled Students' Allowance (DSA) is a non means tested grant that helps with the cost of studying, including equipment, specialist software, or personal assistance.

Many people with spinal injuries find that studying:
- Builds self esteem and confidence
- Opens up new career paths or interests
- Provides mental stimulation and structure
- Creates a focus during long recovery periods

Even short courses, such as photography, learning a language, IT, or counselling - can spark a sense of progress and fulfilment.

Returning to Work or Discovering Something New

Not everyone will return to the job they had before injury, and that is perfectly okay. The journey back into employment may look different for each individual.

Some common routes include:
- Returning to a previous role with reasonable adjustments
- Switching to part-time or remote work
- Retraining in a new field of interest
- Starting a small business or becoming self employed
- Volunteering to rebuild skills and confidence before applying for paid roles

What matters most is that the person feels empowered to choose a path that suits their new reality. For many, working again on their own terms, can bring back a sense of identity, purpose, and self worth.

Support Is Available

There are schemes and organisations specifically designed to help disabled people access work, training, and personal development.

Access to Work (UK Government)

A major support scheme offering practical help for disabled people in employment. This may include:
- Specialist equipment or technology

- Travel-to-work support
- Workplace adaptations
- A personal support worker or assistant
- Mental health support
- Communication assistance for interviews

This support is available even for people who are self-employed or starting a new job.
More information: www.gov.uk/access-to-work

Scope – Support to Work
A free coaching service that offers online and phone support for disabled adults seeking employment.
Website: www.scope.org.uk

Spinal Injuries Association (SIA)
Offers tailored advice about returning to work, changing careers, and understanding employment rights.
Website: www.spinal.co.uk

What About Disclosure?

Many families worry about whether their loved one will need to disclose their spinal injury when applying for work. Legally, disclosure is only required if:

- Reasonable adjustments are needed
- The condition affects the ability to meet essential job requirements
- The role involves safety critical tasks (e.g. driving, emergency services)

However, being open early in the process can help employers understand what support is needed and demonstrates a commitment to clear communication.

The Equality Act 2010 protects disabled people from discrimination in recruitment, employment, and redundancy. Everyone has the right to fair treatment and equal opportunity in the workplace.

Confidence and Pacing

Returning to study or work is not always a smooth road. It takes time, patience, and gradual progress. The person may need to rebuild stamina, adapt to new environments, or learn to manage fatigue. This is all part of the process—and it is okay to go slowly.

Many individuals begin by:
- Volunteering for just a few hours each week
- Taking one online course module
- Working from home part-time
- Starting a phased return to work with a supportive employer

Every step forward counts. There is no set timeline, and progress is personal.

Purpose Can Take Many Forms

Purpose and contribution do not always mean full-time employment. They may come in other, equally meaningful

forms such as:
- Running a small home-based business
- Mentoring others with similar injuries
- Studying a topic that sparks joy or curiosity
- Engaging in creative outlets like writing, art, or music
- Contributing to the community through advocacy or volunteer work

What matters most is that it feels fulfilling to the person living it. As family members and loved ones, your encouragement and belief in their potential, no matter how different life looks now, can make all the difference. Purpose is not lost. It just evolves.

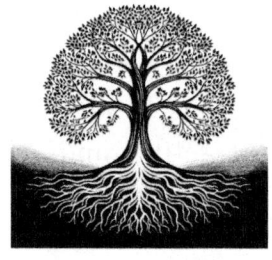

Chapter 10: Emotional Wellbeing, Relationships, and Intimacy After Spinal Injury

Healing the Mind, Heart and Human Connection

Spinal cord injury changes far more than just the body. It can affect identity, confidence, relationships, mental health, and how people connect with themselves and each other. What happens physically is only part of the story - what happens emotionally is equally important and deserving of support.
Yet this is often the part that receives the least attention.
This chapter is here to say: whatever you or your loved one are feeling - grief, confusion, anger, shame, or fear - it is valid. None of this is easy, but none of it is shameful either. The emotional journey after spinal injury is complex, but it is one that can be navigated with care, support, and connection.

The Emotional Crash: When the Reality Sinks In

In the early stages - hospitalisation, surgery, or initial rehabilitation - many people operate in survival mode. There is structure, urgency, questions to answer, and care routines to learn. But as the dust settles and daily life resumes, the emotional impact often begins to surface.

For individuals with spinal cord injury, this may include:
- Grief for the life and body they once had
- Anger at the randomness or unfairness of what happened
- Shame or discomfort around needing help
- Fear about the future, relationships, work, or independence
- A profound loss of control

For families and carers, it can include:
- Shock and trauma from witnessing what happened
- Guilt for feeling tired, angry, or overwhelmed
- Helplessness from not being able to fix things
- Grief for the life or plans that are no longer possible
- Fear of doing something wrong or not being enough

These emotions are not only normal - but they are also expected. The biggest mistake families often make is trying to push past these feelings too quickly. Emotional pain does not disappear when ignored; it needs time, acknowledgment, and honesty to heal.

Mental Health: The Silent Struggle

I know we touched the subject of mental health earlier, but I cannot stress enough how important that is for the individual and their family. Depression, anxiety, and even post traumatic stress are common following spinal cord injury - for the individual, but also for those closest to them. And yet these struggles are often hidden.

Why? Because everyone is trying to stay strong. Because they do not want to worry each other. Because society still treats mental health as a secondary concern.

But mental health is essential. It is not a luxury - it is a vital part of recovery.

One young man I supported had been through more than most people his age. He struggled deeply with feelings of worthlessness. He saw himself as less than - undesirable, burdensome, broken. There were days he asked questions no one wants to hear - questions about suicide. He could not see what others saw. It took time. Honest conversations. Quiet encouragement. We talked about the family who loved him, about the pride his parents felt in how far he had come, about the strength it took to keep getting up and doing the work. I reminded him of what I saw each day - a young man showing up for his physiotherapy, pushing through the discomfort, making visible progress, even in just the short two years I had known him.

He did not wake up one morning transformed. But gradually, he stopped fixating on what was missing or broken, and began to see what remained - and what could still grow.

The Carer's Emotional Load

Caring with love is beautiful - but it must also be sustainable.

Many family members - partners, parents, adult children - step into the role of carer after a spinal injury. Often, this happens instinctively, from a place of love. But when someone becomes the main source of both emotional and physical care, it can affect relationships and wellbeing in profound ways.

Carers often carry:
- Guilt for needing rest, space, or support
- Exhaustion from physical care and emotional vigilance

- Sadness about the relationship changing
- Fear of burnout or making mistakes
- A loss of identity beyond the carer role

You are not a machine. You are allowed to need care, too.

Helpful support may include:
- Professional counselling or therapy (ideally with someone who understands disability or trauma)
- Peer support groups (in-person or online)
- Honest conversations within the family about how each person is coping
- Speaking to a GP or spinal team if mood, appetite, or sleep patterns change
- Medication, if needed and without shame
- Carer support services and respite options

The stronger and more supported you feel, the more loving and sustainable your care can be.

Preserving Relationships and Boundaries

Spinal injury can shift the dynamic between loved ones. Romantic partners may become carers. Parents may struggle to maintain boundaries. Friendships may fade, not out of malice, but because people do not know what to say.

It is easy for relationships to become unbalanced - but they do not have to be. One of the most compassionate and practical steps a family can take is to bring in trained carers or personal assistants. This allows partners to remain partners, parents to be parents, and relationships to stay emotionally connected rather than overwhelmed by care routines.

Professional carers bring:
- Structure and predictability
- Clinical knowledge and physical care experience
- Emotional distance, which creates space for family connection

This does not mean loved ones should step back entirely - but rather that their role can be one of love, presence, and emotional closeness, rather than full time care.

As a carer who has spent most of my career working within family homes, I have seen time and again how easily loved ones - partners, parents, children - can become completely overwhelmed when trying to take on the role of primary carer. The love is never in question, but the exhaustion builds quietly until it begins to affect not just their wellbeing, but the relationship itself.

One mother once confided in me that while she would have done anything for her son, she no longer felt like his mum - she felt like a nurse. A partner once said she missed being a wife, a partner; everything had become about medication, routines, and transfers.

These are painful truths, but they are common.

That is why it is so important to protect the original roles within a relationship - to ensure that loved ones are not forced into becoming sole carers. Involving professional support does not mean caring less. In fact, it often means caring better. It allows family members to be exactly who they are meant to be:

a parent, a partner, a sibling - someone who is emotionally present, not just physically helpful.

Preserving these roles, wherever possible, protects both the person with the injury and those who love them. It allows space for rest, for reconnection, and for relationships to grow beyond the injury - not be defined by it.

Intimacy, Identity and Emotional Connection

Spinal injury does not erase desire. It does not end the need for touch, closeness, or sexual identity. But it does change how these needs are expressed and experienced.

For many people, injury raises difficult questions:
- Will I ever be desired again?
- Can I still be intimate with my partner?
- Will people see my disability before they see me?

These feelings are deeply human - and they are not the end of the story.

Body Image and Confidence

After injury, many people struggle to feel at home in their bodies. Surgical scars, weight changes, catheters, and new routines can all affect confidence. But your body - no matter how it moves or looks - is still worthy of love, comfort, and connection.

Healing body image often begins with:
- Gentle reconnection through daily care or massage

- Wearing clothing that feels good
- Seeing yourself through the eyes of those who love you
- Allowing yourself to be seen, even when vulnerable

Dating After Injury

If you or your loved one is single, the idea of dating after spinal injury can feel overwhelming. There may be fears about rejection, uncertainty about when or how to disclose the injury, or a quiet worry that nobody will see beyond the wheelchair.

But here is the truth: relationships are human. They are built on connection, not perfection. They do not rely on physical ability. And they are absolutely still possible.

I had the privilege of working with one client for many years. Not long after his accident, I read an interview where he had said, "Who would want me now?" At the time, it was a heartbreaking reflection of how lost and unlovable he felt. But a few years later, I witnessed that same man fall in love, begin a relationship, and eventually get engaged. Everything he thought was no longer possible became part of his new life. Not because it fell into his lap, but because he allowed himself to show up - to be seen, to connect and to let someone in.

Relationships may not unfold exactly as they once did - but they can be rich, beautiful, and deeply meaningful. Just like before, they take courage, vulnerability, and presence.

Another client I supported was a university student, living in a dormitory and continuing to date his long-time girlfriend who had been by his side since before the injury. Their relationship did not end because of the accident - it evolved. Together, they adapted, faced challenges, and kept choosing each other.

These stories are reminders that love is not defined by injury. But it does require participation. If someone is hiding away in their bedroom, shielding themselves from the world, then yes - it will feel impossible to meet someone. But when you step out into life again, when you allow others to see your humour, your heart, and your presence, that is when connection becomes possible.

The people who truly matter will see beyond the chair. And they will see you.

Sexuality After Injury

Sex may look different - but it can still be deeply meaningful.

Depending on the level of injury, there may be changes in sensation, arousal, or physical function. But intimacy is not defined by what is lost - it is created through connection, vulnerability, trust, and shared joy.

Support is available:
- Medical teams can advise on medications, aids, and physical adaptations
- Occupational therapists can help with comfort and positioning
- Sexual health specialists and psychosexual therapists can support individuals or couples

You are still deserving of love, desire, and pleasure - however that looks for you now.

Emotional Intimacy and Communication

True closeness is not only physical - it is emotional. It comes from shared vulnerability, laughter, honesty, and care.

For couples navigating injury together:
- Speak openly about needs, fears, and frustrations
- Create time for connection outside of the care routine
- Let go of guilt around shifting roles and focus on rebuilding partnership
- Seek therapy or relationship support if needed

If you are single and navigating dating after injury, remember this: your injury does not define your worth. You bring personality, humour, depth, care, and a body capable of connection. The right people will see you, not just your injury.

In Summary

Emotional wellbeing, relationships, and intimacy are not extras - they are essential. They are part of what makes life meaningful.

Spinal cord injury may change how people connect, express love, or feel about themselves - but it does not take away their humanity. Nor does it erase the deep love and connection that families share.

To those living with injury: You are still you. You are allowed to grieve, to love, to desire, to ask for help, and to rebuild life on your own terms.

To those supporting someone you love: Your care matters. So does your wellbeing. You are allowed to love fiercely and still ask for help.

Healing happens not only in the body - but in the mind, the heart, and the relationships that carry us through.

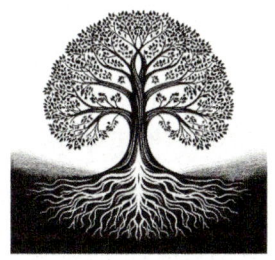

Chapter 11: Parenting and Family Life After Spinal Injury

Still Mum. Still Dad. Still You.

One of the most common and painful fears following a spinal cord injury - especially for those with children, is: "Will I still be able to be there for my child?" Whether they are toddlers needing to be carried or teenagers craving emotional connection, the thought of being absent, physically or emotionally, can weigh heavily on the mind and heart.

But the truth remains: you are still their parent. That role is not taken away by injury. While some of the "how" may change, the love, presence, and ability to nurture and guide your children remain firmly intact.

Rebuilding Your Role as a Parent

Returning home after injury is a significant adjustment - not only for the individual, but for the entire family. Children often adapt more quickly than adults anticipate, but they are perceptive. They notice shifts in mood, routine, and energy, and they benefit immensely from clear, honest communication.

One of my clients had two young nieces who grew up with him using a wheelchair - it was simply part of their world. But when they started preschool and heard questions from other children, they came to him one day curious: "Why don't you walk?" He had the most wonderful, age appropriate way of explaining it. He told them the spinal cord is like a telephone line between the brain and the legs - and his line had been broken. So even though his mind still wanted to tell his legs to walk, the message could not get through. It was simple, honest, and perfectly suited for a child's understanding. And it gave them clarity without fear.

Speaking openly helps children feel safe. You might say:
- "I may need help with some things, but I am still the one who tucks you in."
- "I might do things differently now, but I am still your mum or dad."
- "You do not have to take care of me - we are a team, and I love you."

Restoring familiar routines - like helping with homework, bedtime stories, school runs, or weekend activities, even with adaptations - helps reestablish a parental role in a way that is meaningful and reassuring for the whole family.

Practical Adaptations for Everyday Parenting

Parenting does not have to look the same as before. There are many practical tools and creative solutions that allow continued, confident involvement in your child's life:

- Adaptive equipment such as wheelchair height baby cribs, adjustable changing tables, and modified child car seats

- Transfer aids, lap trays, and lightweight mobility devices for handling daily tasks safely
- Smart home devices, hands free communication tools, and visual aids to support routine and organisation

And just as important - do not hesitate to ask for help when needed. Delegating physical tasks does not diminish your role as a parent. Presence, love, and consistency matter more than perfection.

Supporting Your Partner and Co-Parent

If you are parenting as part of a couple, both people may be adjusting to new roles, responsibilities, and emotional weight. It is essential to support one another not only as co-parents, but as partners.

Be available to:
- Talk honestly about frustrations, fears, and changing routines
- Avoid assumptions - rebuild roles together, not in isolation
- Set aside moments for your relationship, separate from parenting or care responsibilities
- Let children see your teamwork; it builds their emotional security

If you are parenting alone, building a reliable support network - family, friends, care staff - can provide essential backup and emotional space.

Pregnancy and Parenthood After Injury

Spinal injury does not remove the possibility of becoming a parent. Many people go on to have healthy pregnancies and births following injury. With support from spinal consultants, midwives, and obstetric teams, parenthood remains very much within reach.

And for those already raising children, the ability to care has not disappeared. It may require time, adaptations, and creativity - but it is possible.

Children Are Remarkably Resilient

Children are curious, open, and capable of understanding more than they are often given credit for. When included in the process, they often adapt with grace, become strong little advocates, and continue to thrive in a home filled with love.

What children need most is:
- Emotional presence
- Affection and reassurance
- Honest, age appropriate communication
- The comfort of knowing that their parent is still their parent

Your child still wants to tell you their stories, ask you their questions, and run to you when they are hurt or excited. That does not change with mobility aids or medical routines.

Family Life Continues - and Grows

The shape of family life may shift - but the heartbeat remains.

You can still:
- Attend school plays
- Cheer from the sidelines at football matches
- Take family holidays
- Be present at bedtime
- Help with school projects
- Host birthday parties
- Laugh together, cry together, and grow together

Yes, some things may need more planning or support. But your presence continues to be the most important thing.

Different Roles, Same Love

Not everyone raising or loving children after spinal injury is a biological parent.

I worked with one client who did not have children of his own, but who was an exceptional uncle. His nieces absolutely adored him. He was playful, attentive, and completely present - exactly what every child needs from a role model. Another young man I supported had been married for five years before his injury. He and his wife were actively trying for a baby when it happened. Their dream did not disappear - they simply began navigating it with greater support and determination.

Love, guidance, fun and presence - these are the pillars of family life. They are not limited by physical ability.

In Summary

Spinal injury may change the way you parent - but it does not change that you parent. You are still mum. Still dad. Still the source of safety, love, and guidance that your children need.

Your family still needs your voice, your stories, your warmth, and your steady presence - even if it is offered in a new way. You still belong at the heart of your home.

And you have every right to continue growing as a parent, shaping your family's future, and celebrating all the messy, beautiful, ordinary moments that make life rich.

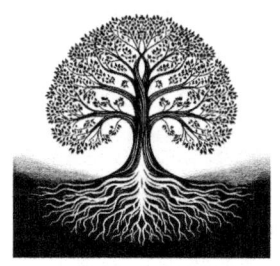

Chapter 12: Finding Support, Building Community, and Staying Connected

You Are Not Alone and You Still Belong

Spinal cord injury does not just affect the body. It introduces a new world - full of appointments, systems, assessments, and unfamiliar acronyms. NHS, ICBs, PIP, OT, MDT suddenly, life feels more like a tangle of paperwork than a path forward. It can be exhausting, overwhelming, and isolating.

But within that complexity, there is help. And beyond the systems and services, there are people. There are communities. There are friends - some old, some new - ready to walk this road with you.

You do not have to do this alone.

Support Is Out There, But You May Need to Speak Up

Many families do not receive the support they are entitled to - not because it does not exist, but because no one tells them how to access it. Or because the process feels too complicated to even begin.

That can and must change.

You do not need to know every form or acronym. But you do need to speak up, stay persistent, and ask questions. Support systems are not always designed to be easy - but they are there. And you deserve to benefit from them.

Accessing Medical, Social and Financial Support

Spinal injury qualifies individuals for a range of long term support services. Some are provided directly through NHS, spinal centres, others through local councils, charities, or national benefits systems. The key is knowing where to look - and asking for help navigating them.

Medical and Rehabilitation Services often include:
- Outreach spinal nurses
- Physiotherapists and occupational therapists
- Bladder, bowel, respiratory, or urology clinics
- Tissue viability teams for skin care
- Lifelong follow-up through spinal units

Ask for:
- A named contact at your spinal unit
- Direct numbers for urgent concerns (e.g. skin breakdown, autonomic dysreflexia)
- Information about review schedules and community integration

Social Care and Equipment Provision through your local council may include:
- Care assessments
- Home adaptations (e.g. ramps, stairlifts, wet rooms)
- Profiling beds, hoists, or mobility equipment
- Direct payments or Personal Health Budgets for managing care

Financial Support and Benefits may include:
- Personal Independence Payment (PIP)
- Carer's Allowance
- Universal Credit or ESA
- Council Tax reduction
- Blue Badge scheme
- Charitable grants

Always get up to date guidance through Citizens Advice, Spinal Injuries Association (SIA), or a local welfare rights advisor. Keep records. Request written assessments. Document all communications.

You Deserve Advocacy

Sometimes, things go wrong. Assessments are denied. Equipment is delayed. Care packages are incomplete. You are well within your rights to:
- Request reassessments
- Appeal decisions
- Ask for a second opinion
- Submit formal complaints
- Work with an advocate who understands the system

Organisations like the Spinal Injuries Association, Beacon, Aspire, and Disability Rights UK can help. You do not have to fight these battles alone.

The Power of Community

Beyond the systems and services lies something just as vital: human connection.

Spinal injury can be isolating. Daily routines become clinical. Social life shrinks. It may feel as if the world has moved on while you have been left behind.

But you are not just a patient. You are not just a care plan.
You are still a friend, neighbour, sibling, teammate, partner. And those roles matter just as much as your physical recovery.

Let People In They Want to Show Up

One of the most beautiful parts of this journey is seeing the good in people - often when you least expect it.

I mentioned this earlier - One of my clients befriended many neighbours simply by going out with his dog, well story did not end there. One day my client became seriously unwell and was taken into hospital by ambulance. Before we had even left the house, neighbours were on the doorstep asking how they could help. Naturally, one of our biggest concerns was his dog - routine, care, exercise. Within a single day, our neighbours had set up a rota. Someone came to feed and let the dog out. Someone else took him for long walks. He was played with, loved, and looked after every day my client was in hospital.
And this was not just once. It happened again and again over the years - each time with no need to ask, no hesitation. Even when he was back home but too weak to take the dog for a walk himself, a neighbour would knock, leash in hand, ready to help.

That kind of support is not luck. It is the result of being willing to open up a little. To be seen. To smile, to stop and talk, to show up in your own street. Because the truth is, people often do want to help - but they cannot help someone they have never had the chance to know.

Those people were not asked. They simply saw a need and responded with kindness.

Another year, on Christmas Eve, we had just finished delivering small gifts to his nieces - a tradition my client never missed. As we were returning home, his wheelchair accessible van broke down. It was freezing, and recovery time was estimated at three hours. His brother reached out to his neighbour - someone who had bonded with my client over their shared love of football, they both were supporting their local team, they would meet at every home game. Without hesitation, that man arranged for a family member to drive his wheelchair accessible van, pick us up, and bring us home. Simply so my client would not be left sitting in the cold.

This is what happens when you let yourself be seen. When you allow others into your life, even in small ways. Communities are not built through grand gestures - they grow through simple acts of connection.

Staying Connected in a Changed World

Isolation is not always physical. Emotional barriers - fear, grief, anxiety about being seen differently - can be just as limiting. But connection is a powerful medicine.

Small steps can rebuild a sense of belonging:
- Join a local or virtual support group
- Volunteer, even a few hours a month
- Attend accessible sports or leisure activities
- Explore peer mentoring through SIA, Back Up Trust, or Aspire

- Stay active in your faith group, community events, or neighbourhood gatherings
- Use online forums and disability communities to stay in touch

You do not have to wait until you "feel ready." Sometimes connection brings readiness.

Friendships May Change - Let Them Evolve

It is true: some friends will fade. Not everyone knows how to navigate change. That can hurt deeply, but it is not a reflection of your worth.

Others will show up more than ever. You will find new connections - people who have been through something similar, or who simply choose to show up with kindness.

Let go of guilt for relationships that drift. Focus on those who lean in.

Getting Involved On Your Own Terms

Being part of a community does not require big commitments. It may look like:
- Helping with a local event from home
- Mentoring someone recently injured
- Campaigning for better access
- Supporting a friend
- Saying hello to neighbours
- Being visible and involved in whatever way feels right

You still have something to offer. You always have something to share.

In Summary

Spinal injury may change the systems you navigate and the way you participate, but it does not erase your place in the world.

You are still entitled to support. You are still part of your community. And when you allow others in, when you reach out, ask for help, and say yes to connection - you do not just improve your own life. You show others that there is life after injury. A life of meaning, purpose, and belonging.

You still matter.
You are not alone.
And you are still part of something bigger.

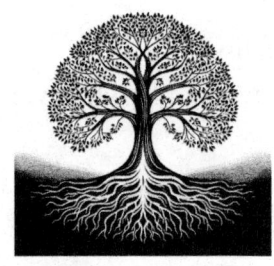

Chapter 13: Travel and Freedom

Reclaiming Independence, Exploring the World and Planning With Confidence

One of the most common myths about spinal cord injury is that life becomes confined to the home. That outings become rare, holidays become impossible, and freedom disappears.

That is simply not true.

Yes, travel after injury requires more planning. But it remains absolutely possible - whether it is a trip to the café, a weekend away, or a flight across the world. With preparation, support, and the right information, movement becomes manageable - and the confidence that follows is life changing.

This chapter is about helping you get out there again. Because your world has not closed - it has simply changed shape.

Getting Around Locally

Daily outings are an important part of reclaiming independence - whether it is running errands, visiting friends, going out for coffee or a meal, or simply attending appointments. Accessible transport and advance preparation can make all the difference. Public transport is accessible and fantastic option if you do not own a vehicle. Also check local taxi or private hire companies so you know where to find accessible taxi when one is needed. Get name and phone number – bit of advice, if you know in advance you will need it – pre book it. They can get busy and you may face long wait time otherwise.

Travelling by Train

Train travel across the UK is possible - and often well supported when planned ahead.

Tips for a smoother journey:
- Book assistance 24+ hours in advance via the train company or National Rail's Passenger Assistance service.
- Request portable ramps, wheelchair spaces, or help at platforms.
- Confirm whether your departure and arrival stations have step-free access.
- Disabled Persons Railcards offer discounts, and carers may qualify for companion tickets.

Travelling by Car

For many, driving or being driven remains the most flexible option for travel.

Key considerations:
- Ensure adapted vehicles have the necessary ramps, hoists, or hand controls.
- Carry a Radar Key and plan rest stops with accessible toilets.

- Register your vehicle for:
  - Vehicle tax exemptions (DVLA)
  - Congestion and ULEZ charge exemptions (TfL)
  - Toll road schemes (e.g. Dartford Crossing, Mersey Gateway)

Registration is often required in advance - Blue Badge eligibility alone does not guarantee exemption. Visit www.gov.uk or local transport authority websites for details.

The Motability Scheme (UK)

For those receiving the enhanced mobility component of PIP or DLA:
- Lease a new car, wheelchair accessible vehicle (WAV), scooter, or powerchair.
- Insurance, servicing, road tax, and breakdown cover are included.
- Adaptations (e.g. hand controls, swivel seats, ramps) may be fitted at no additional cost.

Learn more: www.motability.co.uk

Blue Badge Scheme

Provides parking concessions such as:
- Free or discounted parking
- Access to disabled bays near entrances
- Permission to park on yellow lines (where allowed)

Apply through your local authority or www.gov.uk/apply-blue-badge

Useful Tools and Apps

- AccessAble, Euan's Guide, and Blue Badge Parking UK help check accessibility in advance.
- Always confirm locations for:
  - Disabled parking
  - Step-free entry
  - Accessible toilets (Changing Places or Radar Key)

Air Travel with a Spinal Injury

Flying is absolutely possible - and airlines are legally required to provide assistance.

Before Booking:
- Contact the airline's special assistance team to discuss needs.
- Ask about:
  - Boarding assistance and aisle chairs
  - Wheelchair storage
  - Accessibility of onboard toilets
  - Seating options (bulkhead, extra legroom)
  - Transport of battery-powered chairs or medical supplies

At the Airport:
- Arrive early and check in at the designated assistance desk.
- Carry a pressure relief cushion for long flights.
- Keep essential medication in hand luggage.
- Bring a GP or consultant letter listing all your medication, catheter supplies, mobility equipment and care needs.

- Confirm in advance where you will collect your wheelchair upon arrival. Some airports have policies that allow your wheelchair to be returned to you at the aircraft door, while others may require you to collect it from baggage reclaim.

Tip: Add a label to your wheelchair with handling instructions and contact details. Photograph your chair before flight in case of damage.

Accommodation In the UK or Abroad

Do not rely solely on website descriptions of "accessible." Always call or email to confirm key features:
- Roll in showers or wet rooms
- Lift access or ground floor location
- Bed clearance for hoists
- Door widths and toilet access
- Emergency evacuation plans

Helpful booking platforms include:
- Handiscover
- Euan's Guide
- Many popular hotel chains have accessible rooms (for domestic and international stays)
- Specialist accessible travel agents for cruises or international destinations

Travel Insurance

It is essential to purchase travel insurance that covers pre-existing medical conditions, including spinal cord injury.

Look for policies that:
- Include cover for mobility equipment (e.g. wheelchairs, ventilators)
- Cover carer or personal assistant costs
- Do not exclude common complications (e.g. UTIs, pressure injuries)
- Provide emergency repatriation cover

There is several providers that have policies that will cover person with spinal injury.

Hiring or Renting Equipment While Travelling

If taking all your usual equipment is impractical, you can rent:
- Hoists and slings
- Profiling beds
- Wheelchairs or powerchairs
- Shower chairs, commodes, or pressure relief cushions

Plan well in advance and notify your accommodation provider. There is many companies in UK and all over the world who will rent equipment needed. Check their websites, call them, give them make and model of equipment you are using at home, so they can try to match it, or find replacement as close as possible to the usual equipment.

Planning for the Unexpected

Travel brings joy - but also risk. Being prepared reduces stress.

Carry:
- A copy of your care plan and emergency contacts
- A letter from your GP or spinal consultant
- Spare medical supplies
- A list of nearby hospitals or spinal units (especially abroad)

And always pack with confidence, not fear.

In Summary

Travel after spinal cord injury is not only possible - it is empowering. The first trip may feel daunting, but confidence builds with each outing. Whether it is a short drive, a family visit, or a dream holiday, the world is still open to you.
Your wheels do not hold you back. They carry you forward.

On the next page, you will find a Travel Preparation Checklist, a practical tool to help you feel prepared and supported when travelling.

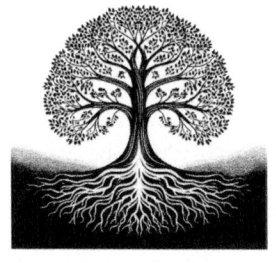

Travel Preparation Checklist

A helpful guide to support your planning and peace of mind when travelling with someone who has care needs.

Local Travel (Car / Train / Bus)
- Blue Badge clearly displayed
- Vehicle registered for congestion or toll exemptions
- RADAR key packed for accessible toilets
- Route checked for accessibility and rest stops
- Rail assistance booked (if applicable)
- Water and snacks packed
- Emergency medication (e.g. Nifedipine, Glyceryl Trinitrate spray)
- Regular medications organised and accessible

Air Travel
- Airline contacted and assistance arranged
- Mobility or medical equipment declared (e.g. battery-powered wheelchair, ventilator)
- Medical documentation (doctor's letter, prescriptions, care notes) packed
- Pressure relief cushion or mattress support included
- Pre-boarding confirmed
- In-flight toilet access discussed with airline
- Medications, including emergency meds, in hand luggage
- Extra water, snacks, and comfort items prepared

Accommodation
- Accessibility confirmed via phone/email (door width, bed height, bathroom access)
- Equipment rental arranged (e.g. hoist, shower chair) if needed
- Accessible parking available
- Evacuation plan discussed and understood
- Fridge access for medication (if required)

Insurance & Documentation
- Specialist travel insurance confirmed (covering medical needs and equipment)
- Copies of:
  - Medical notes and medication list
  - Emergency care plan
  - Passport and ID
  - Translated medical instructions (if travelling abroad)
- Contact details for local emergency services and embassy (if abroad)

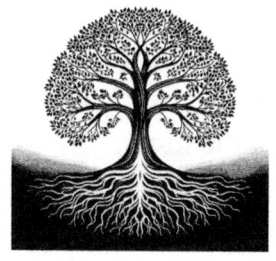

Chapter 14: Life After Injury - Purpose, Resilience and Living Fully

Before we begin, I want to acknowledge that some of what you are about to read may echo points mentioned earlier in this guide. That repetition is intentional. These notes - about purpose, resilience, connection and the power of showing up - are not just important; they are vital. They deserve to be said more than once, because they are the heart of what makes life after spinal injury not only possible, but meaningful and fulfilling.

Because Survival Is Only the Beginning

A spinal cord injury changes far more than the physical body. It reshapes identity, interrupts plans, and challenges everything from relationships to routine. In the beginning, life becomes a blur of survival, adjustment, and loss. But as time moves forward, a new question begins to emerge - sometimes quietly, sometimes with urgency: What now?

This chapter is not here to tell you that everything will return to how it was. It will not. But it is here to say that life continues. That meaning, joy, connection, and legacy are still within reach. That surviving was only the first chapter - and now you are living and writing the rest.

Redefining Identity

Many of my clients describe the early weeks and months after injury as a kind of unraveling. Roles they once knew - parent, worker, athlete, traveller, partner - feel distant or suspended. There is a grief not just for the body, but for the sense of self. But identity is not lost. It is rebuilt.

In time, people discover that who they are is not defined only by movement or independence. With the support of peers, therapy, community, and new experiences, they begin to reclaim themselves - sometimes in ways they never expected.

That might mean:
- Embracing a long neglected passion or hobby
- Becoming an expert in their own care, and teaching others
- Strengthening relationships that matter most
- Discovering patience, empathy, or perspective that could only come through adversity

Life does not shrink unless you let it, it evolves. That evolution can be extraordinary.

Resilience Is Not a Slogan - It Is a Way of Living

Real resilience is not about staying strong at all times. It is about continuing, even when everything feels fragile. It is recognising your own limits and honouring them. It is laughing, even on hard days. It is choosing to show up - again and again - for your life.

Resilience might look like:
- Taking the day slowly, because that is what your body needs
- Asking for help without shame
- Letting go of things that no longer serve you
- Starting over, even after a setback

It is not about pretending. It is about being real. And in being real, you become remarkably strong.

Returning to Work - Or Finding Purpose in New Ways

Not everyone returns to employment after spinal injury, and that is entirely valid. For some, the medical or logistical complexity is simply too great. But for others, the journey back to work is both possible and empowering.

Support is available:
- Access to Work grants
- Inclusive employers with reasonable adjustments
- Flexible and remote working options
- Vocational rehabilitation and career re-training

But purpose does not depend on a payslip. Fulfilment can be found in:
- Volunteering
- Mentoring someone newly injured
- Sharing your story to educate and advocate
- Starting a personal project or campaign

One client of mine experienced a life-changing injury while "tombstoning"- jumping from a height into shallow sea water. It happened in seconds, but it altered everything. In the years that followed, he became a respected voice in his community, using his story to raise awareness of water safety. He appeared in interviews, public service campaigns, and even spoke in schools. He once told me, "If sharing my story stops one person from doing what I did - it is worth it."

That is purpose. That is legacy in real time.

Parenting, Family Life, and Emotional Closeness

Yes, parenting is still possible. So is dating, becoming a grandparent, being a role model, and creating a home filled with laughter and connection. Family life changes - but it continues.

I have seen clients:
- Read bedtime stories from their wheelchairs
- Push prams using adaptive attachments
- Be the loudest voice at school plays or football games
- Remain the safe space their children return to, no matter what

Children are often the quickest to adapt. They see love before they see difference. And they care far more about presence than perfection.

Family life may look different - but it can become even more rooted in emotional presence, teamwork, and shared joy.

Creativity, Hobbies, and Adaptive Sport

Injury often opens doors to creativity. With routines changed, people make space for art, music, writing, photography, and nature. Hobbies become both therapy and expression. An adaptive sport has transformed thousands of lives.

Through organisations like WheelPower and Back Up Trust, people explore:
- Wheelchair rugby or basketball
- Adaptive skiing or hand-cycling
- Para-swimming or archery
- Sailing, dancing, or simply playing catch with their children

These activities are about more than fitness. They are about empowerment, taking back control, building confidence and having fun.

Joy Still Happens - Laughter Still Comes

One of the greatest fears I hear from newly injured clients is that life will become dull, joyless, or heavy. But after nearly two decades in this work, I can assure you: joy still comes. Often, unexpectedly.

I have seen clients:
- Laugh with their carers about hoist mishaps
- Race their power chair agains their kids bikes with delight and so much laughter
- Celebrate a successful bowel routine with humour and pride

Joy is in the everyday: a café visit, a shared joke, a football match with friends.

One client of mine, a fiercely devoted football fan, continued to attend every home game in his power chair. Rain or shine, he wore his team's colours, knew every chant, and greeted stewards by name. That stadium remained his second home. It gave him rhythm, joy and belonging. He was unstoppable!

I have been with my clients to live gigs, cinemas, theatre performances, tv program recordings of their favourite shows and many, many more events. I travelled in the UK and abroad. Simply because they choose to live fully and not to allow their disability disable them.
I will say this to you – **BE UNSTOPPABLE!**

Living Fully, Even Through the Hard Days

Not every day will be easy. There will be dips, medical setbacks, and moments of grief. But there will also be:
- Deep relationships
- New things to learn and teach
- Laughter that surprises you
- Days that start small and end beautifully

You do not have to be ready for everything. You just have to be present. Living fully means showing up for your life - your way, at your pace.

Your Legacy Is Already Being Written

Legacy is not about wealth or fame. It is about presence. It is in:
- The way you make others feel
- The resilience you model

- The conversations you start
- The quiet courage you show every single day

By living fully - through all of it - you are teaching others what real strength looks like. You are changing lives simply by being here.

In Summary

Life after spinal injury is not a return - it is a reinvention. It is about building something new out of what was lost. And that process takes strength, tenderness, and time.

You are still here. Still becoming. Still offering the world your insight, your humour, your humanity.

Your story did not end with injury. It began again.

And every chapter that follows is yours to write - with purpose, with courage, and with joy.

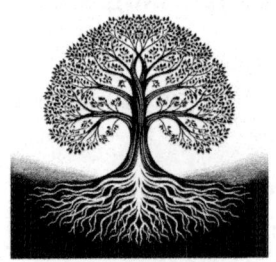

Chapter 15: Planning for the Future

Security, Stability and Confidence for What Comes Next

Before we begin, let us say this clearly: planning for the future is not giving up. It is not negative thinking. It is not a lack of hope. It is courage in its most practical form. It is a way to say, "When the time comes, I want to be heard." And it is one of the most respectful and empowering things you can do- if you choose to - for yourself, and for those who care for you.

This chapter may repeat some messages you have heard already - about clarity, preparation, and the importance of having a voice. That is intentional. These are not ideas to hear once and forget. They are vital. They deserve space.

Thinking Ahead Does Not Mean Letting Go

After spinal injury, so much of life becomes focused on adapting to the moment - on surviving, recovering, stabilising. But when the initial dust settles, it becomes time to look ahead. Planning does not mean defeat. It is about strength. It is about owning your future, creating peace of mind, and ensuring that your needs, values, and wishes are never overlooked.

Whether you are just beginning this journey or have lived with injury for years, it is never too early - or too late - to begin thinking ahead.

Housing and Long Term Living

Some people remain in their original homes long term. Others need to make changes due to stairs, door widths, or unmanageable layouts. This is not failure it is logistics. It is safety and dignity.

Options to consider:
- Moving to a bungalow or accessible flat
- Registering for adapted housing with your local council
- Exploring housing association or supported living schemes

Housing OTs (Occupational Therapists) can assess your needs and support rehousing applications.

Care Planning That Adapts With You

Your care needs may increase. Or decrease. You may rely on family now, but plan to bring in professional support later. Care should not be a fixed idea. It should grow with you
.
Strong, future focused care includes:
- Keeping care plans and emergency protocols updated
- Creating backup care arrangements (for illness or absence)
- Planning for live in or agency care if family support becomes unsustainable
- Regular care reviews to reassess your needs

If you employ Personal Assistants (PAs) through Direct Payments:
- Keep clear contracts and payroll records
- Ensure liability insurance is in place
- Prepare for recruitment or cover if staff leave unexpectedly

Planning is not assuming the worst - it is making sure no one is left scrambling when life shifts.

Financial Planning - Because Security Is Freedom

Living with spinal injury often comes with hidden costs: equipment, maintenance, accessible transport, adaptations, private therapies. It can add up fast.

It is not selfish to want financial stability. It is responsible. It protects your independence and reduces stress for your family.
Steps to take:
- Claim all benefits you are entitled to (PIP, UC, housing support)
- Keep a record of disability related expenses
- Review insurance policies - mobility equipment, home, and life cover
- Set a realistic budget that includes emergency funds

Speak to:
- Welfare rights advisors (Citizens Advice, SIA, Turn2Us)
- Financial advisors with disability planning expertise

Money cannot fix everything - but it can make life easier, calmer, and more flexible.

Legal Planning - Because Your Voice Matters

Legal planning is not just for older adults. It is for anyone who wants control, clarity, and dignity.

Essential tools include:
- Lasting Power of Attorney (LPA): Allows someone you trust to make decisions about your health, finances, or care if you are ever unable to
- Advance Decision to Refuse Treatment (ADRT); A legal document outlining treatments you would decline, such as ventilation or CPR
- Advance Statement: A letter explaining what matters to you - spiritually, emotionally, personally - even if not legally binding
- A Will: Ensures your money, belongings, and final wishes are handled according to your values and priorities

Some people also choose to discuss a Do Not Resuscitate (DNR) decision with their doctors. This is not about giving up. It is about preventing interventions that you feel would be harmful or undignified in specific circumstances.

These are hard conversations. But they are easier now, when everyone is calm, clear, and empowered - than in a moment of crisis. and they are important to have, regardless of what your wishes and plans are. It is important that loved ones are aware of your wishes and preferences.

Planning for Hospital Stays

Even if you are stable now, hospital visits may happen again - planned or emergency. Having a plan in place makes a difficult time safer, smoother, and less stressful.

Create a hospital plan that includes:
- A list of your care needs (bladder, bowel, mobility, transfers, positioning, AD risk)
- Medication lists and allergy details
- Names of key contacts (GP, spinal consultant, family, care manager)
- Emergency protocols (e.g. how you manage autonomic dysreflexia)

Keep this plan:
- In your hospital bag
- With your care team
- Uploaded to digital medical records if possible

Some families laminate it and keep copies in the home and car. In an emergency, clarity can save time - and lives.

It Is Okay to Talk About Death

Spinal injury brings people close to thoughts of mortality. Some push them aside. Others confront them head on.

There is no right way to feel - but there is strength in facing it.
One of my clients chose to sign a DNR after thoughtful discussion with his GP and trusted District Nurse. He said, "I have fought hard to live - but if I am ever at a point where treatment would take away everything I value, I want to be allowed to rest with dignity."

This choice does not mean giving up on life. It means defining what life means for you - and having the courage to name it.

Legacy Is Not About Leaving - It is About Living Now

One client I supported sustained a life changing spinal cord injury and faced a long, emotionally draining legal battle to secure compensation and access to the support she needed. Throughout that process, she became acutely aware of how poorly some professionals - particularly legal representatives - understood the reality of living with spinal injury. The lack of empathy and insight was not just frustrating; it was harmful.

She decided that needed to change. And she chose to be part of that change.

Despite everything she had been through, she began studying law - determined to one day advocate for others in similar situations. She wanted to stand beside people who felt overwhelmed, unheard and ensure that their experience was not dismissed or reduced to paperwork.

That is legacy. It is not about wealth or fame. It is about truth, impact, and using your voice to make things better for someone else. Even when you are still rebuilding your own life.

And yours is already growing.

In Summary

Planning for the future is not morbid. It is powerful.

It protects your rights. It reduces stress for the people who love you. It turns uncertainty into structure. It creates peace of mind. And it lets you focus more of your energy on living, because you have already honoured what comes next.

There is dignity in preparing.

There is love in making things easier for others.

There is courage in saying, "When that time comes, I want it done my way."

And there is life to live - fully, meaningfully, and bravely - until then.

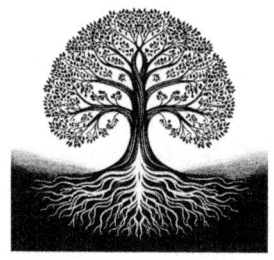

Closing Words: A Letter of Gratitude and Hope

Dear Reader,

Thank you for walking through these pages with me. Whether you read this book in quiet moments at home, in the waiting room of a hospital, or late at night when worry kept you awake, I want you to know how deeply I respect the strength it took to seek out support and understanding.

If you needed this book, it means your life, or the life of someone you love, has been changed by spinal injury. That alone is no small thing. It brings change, challenge and so many unknowns. But it also brings out something remarkable in people: resilience, love, courage, and an ability to adapt that cannot be taught - only lived.

I hope these chapters offered you more than just information. I hope they reminded you that you are not alone. That others have walked this path and continue walking it - sometimes stumbling, sometimes standing strong, but always moving forward in their own way.

This journey is not easy. It is not fair. But it is not hopeless. Even in the hardest moments, there are still connections to be made, small joys to hold on to, and reasons to keep going.

If no one has told you this lately: you are doing an incredible job. Whether you are caring for someone, learning to live with your own injury, or simply holding everything together day by day - that matters. And it is seen.

I wrote this book from my years of experience, but it is your story that brings it to life. However your journey unfolds from here, I hope you carry with you this truth: you are capable, you are needed, and there is still so much ahead that can be meaningful, beautiful, and yours.

I will say it again, if you ever want to reach out - whether to ask a question, share your story, or just vent to someone who understands - you're welcome to email me at:
talktoanna@pm.me

I cannot promise instant answers, but I promise I will read what you write with care.

With all my gratitude and belief in your strength,
Anna

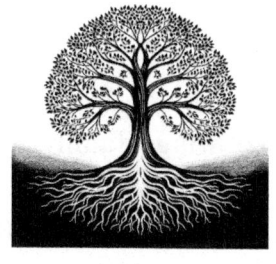

Resources and Further Support

Because You Should Never Have to Do This Alone

This book may be coming to a close, but your journey is still unfolding. And while no guide can anticipate every challenge, one thing remains certain: you should never have to figure it all out by yourself.

Support exists - practical, emotional, financial, medical, and legal. It is out there, and it is for you.

So this chapter is not about closure. It is about connection. About putting the right tools in your hands. About giving you names, numbers, and organisations that can walk with you through whatever comes next.

Because courage is powerful. But it is even more powerful when it is supported.

Spinal Cord Injury Support & Advocacy

Spinal Injuries Association (SIA)
Peer support, legal advocacy, benefits advice, and a free helpline. They also have amazing team of spinal nurses who can help and advise when everything else fails.
www.spinal.co.uk Freephone: 0800 980 0501

Back Up Trust
Wheelchair skills, mentoring, family resources, and youth support.
www.backuptrust.org.uk Tel: 020 8875 1805

Aspire
Grants, adapted housing, assistive tech, and independent living advice.
www.aspire.org.uk Tel: 020 8954 5759

Care Funding and Continuing Healthcare

Integrated Care Boards (ICBs) - formerly known as NHS Continuing Healthcare (CHC) - are responsible for arranging fully funded care packages for people with long term, complex health needs.

For those with spinal injuries, especially where care needs are health related and ongoing, this may mean:
- Integrated Care Boards (ICBs): Full funding for health and personal care, including at home
- Funded Nursing Care (FNC): Support for nursing care in a care home setting
- Personal Health Budget (PHB): Direct funding to manage your own care team or support arrangements

You can request an assessment through your GP, social worker, or spinal unit. This is your right and it can make a world of difference.

Beacon ICB Advice Service
Independent experts offering:
- Free 90-minute advice calls
- Appeals support
- Help navigating the ICB assessment process

www.beaconchc.co.uk | Tel: 0345 548 0300

NHS Information
How to find your local ICBs.
   https://www.nhs.uk/nhs-services/find-your-local-integrated-care-board/

Mental Health & Emotional Support

Mind
Mental health guidance, therapy options, and crisis support.
www.mind.org.uk | Info Line: 0300 123 3393

Samaritans
24/7 free support for anyone feeling overwhelmed or in emotional crisis.
www.samaritans.org | Call: 116 123

CALM (Campaign Against Living Miserably)
Support for men and young people facing suicidal thoughts or depression.
www.thecalmzone.net | Helpline: 0800 58 58 58

Shout (Text Support)
Confidential mental health support via text.
Text SHOUT to 85258

Financial, Legal & Benefits Advice

Citizens Advice
Free guidance on benefits, debt, housing, employment, and legal rights.
www.citizensadvice.org.uk

Turn2Us
Help with benefits checks, grants, and budgeting.
www.turn2us.org.uk

Disability Rights UK
Guidance on benefits, education, independent living, and disability rights.
www.disabilityrightsuk.org

Scope
Support for disabled people with money, employment, and daily life.
www.scope.org.uk | Helpline: 0808 800 3333

Legal Planning & End-of-Life Rights

Office of the Public Guardian (OPG)
For setting up Lasting Power of Attorney (LPA) and understanding your legal rights.
www.gov.uk/power-of-attorney

Compassion in Dying
Advance Decisions (ADRT), end-of-life planning, and support for making your wishes known.
www.compassionindying.org.uk | Advice Line: 0800 999 2434

Age UK
Legal planning, benefits advice, and end-of-life support for older adults and their carers.
www.ageuk.org.uk | Advice Line: 0800 678 1602

Mobility, Travel & Equipment

Motability Scheme
Use your mobility allowance to lease a car, WAV, scooter, or powerchair.
www.motability.co.uk

AccessAble
Check accessibility of public places—hotels, venues, shops, and services.
www.accessable.co.uk

Help with accommodation:
- Handiscover: https://www.handiscover.com
- Euan's Guide: https://www.euansguide.com

Mobility Equipment Hire:

- Rent hoists, beds, commodes, or chairs for UK or international travel. www.mobilityequipmenthiredirect.com
- NRS Healthcare / Millbrook HealthcareSuppliers of NHS and private mobility equipment and daily living aids. www.nrshealthcare.co.uk www.millbrook-healthcare.co.uk

Carers & Family Support

Carers UK
Support, forums, legal advice, and respite care guidance.
www.carersuk.org | Advice Line: 0808 808 7777

The Mix
Support for young carers and young adults under 25.
www.themix.org.uk

YoungMinds
Mental health support for children, teens, and families.
www.youngminds.org.uk

And Finally...
No list is never truly complete, because needs are as individual as the people who live them. But this chapter is a place to start. A quiet reminder that help exists. That there are people who care. That the journey does not need to be walked alone.

Whether you are a person with a spinal injury, a partner, a parent, a friend, or a carer: you deserve support. You deserve peace of mind. And you deserve to know where to turn when things get hard.

Keep this list. Share it. Come back to it. Because even in the hardest chapters, help is still available - and hope is never far away.

The following pages have been intentionally left blank for your use. Whether you wish to note down questions for a consultant, record important details, jot a thought, or keep track of something to follow up - these pages are here for you to use. Sometimes, having a space to write things down can make a real difference. Let these pages be whatever you need them to be.

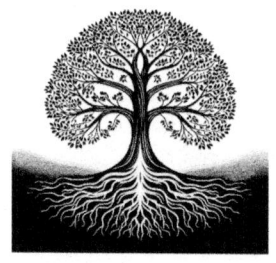

Printed in Dunstable, United Kingdom